STUDY GUIDE FOR

MEDICAL-SURGICAL NURSING

LeMone, Burke, Bauldoff, Gubrud

STUDY GUIDE FOR
MEDICAL-SURGICAL NURSING

Clinical Reasoning in Patient Care

SIXTH EDITION

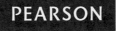

Boston Columbus Indianapolis New York San Francisco Hoboken
Amsterdam Cape Town Dubai London Madrid Milan Munich Paris Montreal Toronto
Delhi Mexico City Sao Paulo Sydney Hong Kong Seoul Singapore Taipei Tokyo

Publisher: Julie Levin Alexander
Publisher's Assistant: Regina Bruno
Product Manager: Pamela Fuller
Development Editor: Pamela Lappies
Editorial Assistant: Erin Sullivan
Project Manager: Cathy O'Connell
Program Manager: Erin Rafferty
Production Editor: Vinolia Benedict Fernando, S4Carlisle Publishing Services
Manufacturing Buyer: Maura Zaldivar-Garcia
Art Director: Maria Guglielmo
Cover Designer: Mary Siener
Interior Design: Ilze Lemesis
Director of Marketing: David Gesell
Senior Product Marketing Manager: Phoenix Harvey
Field Marketing Manager: Debi Doyle
Marketing Specialist: Michael Sirinides
Composition: S4Carlisle Publishing Services
Printer/Binder: Edwards Brother Malloy BAR/Jackson
Cover Printer: Edwards Brothers Malloy BAR/Jackson
Cover Image: David Muir/Getty Images

Credits and acknowledgments borrowed from other sources and reproduced, with permission, in this textbook appear on appropriate page within text.

Notice: Care has been taken to confirm the accuracy of information presented in this book. The authors, editors, and the publisher, however, cannot accept any responsibility for errors or omissions or for consequences from application of the information in this book and make no warranty, express or implied, with respect to its contents.

The authors and publisher have exerted every effort to ensure that drug selections and dosages set forth in this text are in accord with current recommendations and practice at time of publication. However, in view of ongoing research, changes in government regulations, and the constant flow of information relating to drug therapy and drug reactions, the reader is urged to check the package inserts of all drugs for any change in indications of dosage and for added warnings and precautions. This is particularly important when the recommended agent is a new and/or infrequently employed drug.

10 9 8 7 6 5 4 3 2 1

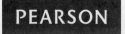

ISBN-10:   0-13-398505-9
ISBN-13: 978-0-13-398505-4

PREFACE

Students entering the field of nursing have a tremendous amount to learn in a very short time. This Study Guide that accompanies *Medical-Surgical Nursing: Clinical Reasoning in Patient Care*, **6th Edition** is designed to reinforce the knowledge that you—the student—have gained in each chapter and to help you master the critical concepts.

Each chapter includes a variety of questions and activities to help you comprehend difficult concepts and reinforce basic knowledge gained from textbook reading assignments. Following is a list of features included in this edition that will enhance your learning experience:

- **Matching** exercises that contain key terms and definitions from each chapter.
- Thorough assessment of essential information in the text is provided through the **Fill in the Blank** activities.
- Multiple-choice **Review Questions** that provide you with additional review on key topics.
- More exercises in the **Focused Study** section.
- **Case Studies** and **Care Plans** that apply concepts from the textbook to real nursing scenarios.
- **Short Answer** exercises that help you learn and retain anatomy and physiology terminology by labeling illustrations from the text and populating tables.

The Answer Key for this Study Guide is posted for easy access on the student resources space for the textbook. By posting these online, we hope to encourage you to critically think through the exercises in this workbook before checking your progress against our suggested answers. You can locate the downloadable Answer Key at www.pearsonhighered .com/nursingresources.

It is our hope that this Study Guide will serve as a valuable learning tool and will contribute to your success in the nursing profession.

CONTENTS

Medical-Surgical Nursing in the 21st Century

LEARNING OUTCOMES

1. Describe the core competencies for healthcare professionals: patient-centered care, interprofessional teams, evidence-based practice, quality improvement, safety, and health information technology.

2. Describe emerging new roles and responsibilities for nurses in an era of healthcare reform.

3. Apply the attitudes, mental habits, and skills necessary for clinical reasoning when using the nursing process in patient care.

4. Explain the importance of nursing and interprofessional codes of ethics and standards of practice as guidelines for clinical nursing practice.

5. Explain the activities and characteristics of the nurse as caregiver, educator, advocate, leader and manager, and researcher.

CLINICAL COMPETENCIES

1. Demonstrate clinical reasoning and apply critical-thinking skills when using the nursing process to provide knowledgeable, safe, patient-centered care.

2. Use health systems technology to provide evidence-based, patient-centered care in all healthcare delivery settings.

3. Provide clinical care that integrates the medical-surgical nursing roles of caregiver, educator, advocate, leader/manager, and researcher.

4. Contribute nursing knowledge and expertise as a member of the interprofessional team to provide safe, quality, and affordable patient-centered care.

TERMS MATCHING

Place the letter of the correct definition in the space next to each term.

1. _____ accountable care organization (ACO)

2. _____ care bundle

3. _____ clinical reasoning

4. _____ code of ethics

5. _____ core competencies

6. _____ critical thinking

7. _____ delegation

8. _____ dilemma

9. _____ ethics

10. _____ health information technology (HIT)

11. _____ health literacy

12. _____ medical-surgical nursing

13. _____ nursing process

14. _____ nursing-sensitive quality indicators (NSQIs)

15. _____ patient

16. _____ patient-centered medical home (PCMH)

17. _____ Patient Protection and Affordable Care Act (ACA)

18. _____ professional boundaries

19. _____ quality improvement

20. _____ standard

21. _____ transitional care

22. _____ Triple Aim

A. Standards that a profession agrees are essential for a person to be deemed competent in his or her field

B. A choice between two unpleasant, ethically troubling alternatives

C. A statement or criterion that can be used by a profession and by the general public to measure quality of practice

D. Health promotion, healthcare, and illness care of adults based on knowledge derived from the arts and sciences and shaped by knowledge of nursing

E. Nursing care is designed and implemented for this person, family, or community

F. A healthcare plan that has been designed with a multidisciplinary, managed care focus

G. To effectively assign appropriate work activities to other members of the healthcare team

H. An established and agreed-on group of principles of conduct that provide a frame of reference for nursing behaviors that are congruent with professional values

I. A series of critical-thinking and clinical-reasoning activities that nurses use as they provide care to patients

J. Self-directed thinking that is focused on what to believe or do in a specific situation

K. Outcomes affected by the quality and quantity of nursing care

L. System designed to promote free exchanges of health information while protecting patients' privacy and improving safety, efficacy, and quality of care

M. Systematic evidence-based methods used to evaluate and improve patient care

N. Accessible, comprehensive, and coordinated primary care focused on illness prevention for patients and families

O. Principles of conduct

P. A complex process that uses cognition, metacognition, and discipline-specific knowledge to gather and analyze patient information, evaluate its significance, and weigh alternative actions

Q. Interventions designed to improve the ability of patients and caregivers to manage care needs in preparation for transitions from one healthcare setting to another or to home

R. An organization aimed at providing accessible, comprehensive and coordinated primary care focused on illness prevention for patients and families

S. A small set of evidence-based interventions for a defined patient population and care setting aimed at improving patient outcomes

T. The degree to which individuals have the capacity to obtain, process, communicate, and understand basic health information and services needed to make appropriate health decisions

U. Borders between the vulnerability of the patient and the power of the nurse

V. Initiative to improve the patient care experience, to maximize positive outcomes, and to contain costs

W. Landmark federal legislation enacted in 2010 and designed to provide access to healthcare services for more Americans and create new models of health care

FOCUSED STUDY

1. Contact your local state board of nursing and request a copy of the nurse practice act. Review the information regarding student nurses.

2. List the five stages of the nursing process. Briefly explain each stage and provide an example of how you may be able to apply each stage of the nursing process in the clinical setting.

   _____

   _____

   _____

   _____

   _____

3. Use your web browser to go to http://www.nursingworld.org/ethics. Describe how the information presented on this site compares to your thoughts about the practice of nursing.

   _____

   _____

   _____

   _____

   _____

CASE STUDY

A 68-year-old female patient has been diagnosed with lung cancer that has metastasized throughout her body. The patient has been admitted to an oncology unit. She has been experiencing an increased amount of pain, and her family has been requesting intravenous morphine for pain control. The patient's respiratory rate has decreased to 9 per minute, but she is still acting as if she's experiencing pain. The physician wrote a p.r.n. order for intravenous morphine that allows the nurses to administer more of the medication per each dose.

1. How might this constitute an ethical dilemma for the nursing staff?

2. What role(s) might the nurse play in helping the patient and the family at this time?

3. How does the code of ethics apply to this patient?

4. Identify two activities the nurse could appropriately delegate to unlicensed personnel in caring for this patient.

5. The patient has become confused and lethargic. What are two nursing concerns that might apply to this patient?

SHORT ANSWERS

Models of Care Delivery

1. Name one type of unit that uses primary nursing as its model of care delivery.

   _____

2. Name one type of unit or facility that uses team nursing as its model of care delivery.

   _____

REVIEW QUESTIONS

1. Which nursing activity occurs as part of the patient assessment in the nursing process?
   1. developing nursing diagnoses
   2. clarifying subjective data
   3. developing a patient care plan
   4. evaluating patient goals

2. The nurse has determined that the patient has not met the outcome criteria that were established 1 month ago. Which actions could the nurse reasonably perform at this time? **Select all that apply.**
   1. Modify the nursing diagnosis.
   2. Modify the outcomes.
   3. Terminate the nursing care plan.
   4. Continue with the nursing care plan.
   5. Modify the nursing care plan.

3. The nurse is dealing with a patient who is very sick. The nurse requires help from an unlicensed staff member to help meet the needs of the nurse's other patients. Which statement by the nurse is most accurate regarding delegation?
   1. "I realize that I am ultimately accountable for the patient's bath."
   2. "As long as I ensure that the unlicensed staff member understands my directions, I can safely allow this person to perform any nursing duty."
   3. "If the unlicensed staff member has been trained to perform this task, I shouldn't be expected to answer any questions that he or she has about the task."
   4. "When I delegate a task, I should be present to watch the task being completed."

4. The nurse is using critical-thinking skills to solve a problem. Which statement best describes *reasoning*?
   1. "I've been weighing the data about the patient's hypertension with the information provided to me about the medications the patient is currently taking."
   2. "I think the patient is really anxious right now, and that's why the patient's apical heart rate is elevated."
   3. "The last time I cared for a patient with a blood pressure this high, the patient had a myocardial infarction."
   4. "I've been thinking about this situation, and I believe there are two possible solutions to the patient's problem."

5. The nurse is performing an assessment on the patient. Which piece of information is subjective?
   1. The patient's blood pressure is 142/78.
   2. The patient states that his pain level is a 4 on a scale of 0–10.
   3. The patient's pupils are dilated.
   4. The patient's right knee is erythematous and edematous.

6. The nurse is documenting information about the patient's assessment. Which piece of documentation indicates that the nurse requires further education?
   1. "Patient is resting quietly in bed."
   2. "Patient was really mean to her husband after the evening meal."
   3. "Patient refused the ordered antiemetic and stated, 'I cannot stay awake when you give me that medication.'"
   4. "Patient turned to the right side and repositioned with pillows."

7. The nurse is providing care for a patient based on the facility's established nursing care plan. Which statement indicates that the nurse requires further education about implementing interventions?
   1. "We need to get your bath done right now, but I'll be back later to look at the incision on your abdomen."
   2. "I'm going to show you how to give yourself the insulin injection right now, but the next time you need one, we'll see how much of this you can do."
   3. "I'll be back in a little while because I need to make notes in your chart about the dressing change to your foot."
   4. "It's really good to see your blood pressure coming down with the medication, and I hope it will be within a normal range by tomorrow."

8. The nurse is educating another less experienced nurse about the rules associated with health information privacy. Which statement by the nurse is inaccurate?
   1. "At times, we have posted a patient's name outside his or her room."
   2. "We must have consent from the patient before we disclose any health information."
   3. "When an older patient has been abused, we must report it."
   4. "At certain times, we have to talk to family members about a patient's care."

Informatics and Evidence-Based Practice in Medical-Surgical Nursing

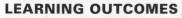

LEARNING OUTCOMES

1. Identify the role of nursing informatics in nursing care.
2. Describe the role of information technology such as computers and related software in nursing care.
3. Define evidence-based practice (EBP).
4. Identify the components of EBP.
5. Describe internal evidence and patient preferences in relationship to EBP.
6. List important citation sources used to locate appropriate external evidence.
7. Compare and contrast the steps of the nursing and evidence-based practice processes.
8. Discuss the role of information technology in the evidence-based practice process.
9. Describe the essential steps of the research process and common statistical methods used in nursing evidence.
10. Describe common steps to implementing EBP in medical-surgical nursing.
11. Discuss ethical considerations in EBP.

CLINICAL COMPETENCIES

1. Demonstrate correct use of computers in the planning and documentation of nursing care.
2. Assess nursing care for evidence basis.
3. Demonstrate correct steps in identifying and locating literature that provides practice evidence.
4. Use common EBP steps used to implement evidence-based practice.
5. Apply ethical behaviors when implementing evidence-based practice interventions.

TERMS MATCHING

Place the letter of the correct definition in the space next to each term.

1. _____ applicability
2. _____ appraisal
3. _____ association
4. _____ causation
5. _____ computer literacy
6. _____ conceptual variable
7. _____ dependent variable
8. _____ descriptive statistics
9. _____ electronic medical records (EMRs)
10. _____ evidence-based practice (EBP)
11. _____ external evidence
12. _____ independent variable
13. _____ inferential statistics
14. _____ information literacy
15. _____ information technology (IT)
16. _____ internal evidence
17. _____ nursing informatics
18. _____ operational variable
19. _____ patient preferences
20. _____ PICOT
21. _____ qualitative research
22. _____ quantitative research
23. _____ reliability
24. _____ research design
25. _____ statistical analysis
26. _____ validity

A. The presumed effect from the manipulation of the independent variable

B. Indicates a relationship only, not cause and effect in research

C. A relationship in which cause and effect are determined

D. Focuses on the extrapolation of research findings to a specific patient situation

E. Familiarity and skills to use a computer

F. Making clinical decisions on the basis of the best available current research evience, clinical expertise, and the needs and preferences of the patient

G. Defines the qualities of the variable of interest in research

H. How well research findings can be applied to specific patient care

I. Statistics used to depict variations within a data set

J. Electronic repository of all patient-related information

K. Relevant research findings related to a specified clinical question

L. A type of evidence used in evidence-based practice that includes nursing expertise and results of quality improvement and outcome evaluations

M. Ability to locate, evaluate, and use appropriate information effectively

N. Format for evidence-based practice question in the form of a mnemonic

O. Uses numerical computations and statistical analysis to answer empirical questions

P. Variable that is manipulated (commonly an intervention)

Q. The mechanical infrastructure that supports the collection, recording, and utilization of patient information

R. Statistics based on the laws of probability

S. A specialty that integrates nursing science, computer science, and information science

T. Serves as a blueprint for conducting a research study

U. Individualized patient experiences and values that are considered when determining evidence-based nursing care

V. Describes the findings of a research study. When used with "instrument," refers to the consistency of the measurement of the variable

W. The manipulation and testing of data from a quantitative study to determine if changes seen are due to the experiment or due to chance

X. A description of how a research variable is measured

Y. Focuses on the participant's experience and the perceived meaning of the situation of interest

Z. The soundness of the scientific methods used in a study

FOCUSED STUDY

1. What was the purpose of TIGER?

_____

_____

_____

_____

_____

2. A major use of information technology involves the documentation of nursing care. What are others uses of information technology in nursing?

_____

_____

_____

_____

_____

3. Identify and explain the four levels of nurse informatics expertise.

_____

_____

_____

_____

_____

4. Describe why nurses should use EBP.

_____

_____

_____

_____

CASE STUDY

Joseph Charles is a nurse researcher interested in learning more about what motivates patients to wait several hours for care in the emergency department when a minor emergency clinic is located two blocks from the hospital. Mr. Charles elects to design a study that will include talking to patients about their decision and the outcome of their emergency department visit.

1. Mr. Charles is investigating research approaches. List and explain the two most common approaches.

2. Mr. Charles elects to use a qualitative approach to this study. List and explain the three major methodologies used in this approach.

3. What questions should Mr. Charles consider regarding the ethics of this study?

SHORT ANSWERS

Complete the following table comparing quantitative and qualitative research.

Quantitative Research	Qualitative Research
Develop research problem.	
	Review related literature. (_Note:_ Not done by all qualitative researchers.)
	Develop overall approach.
Design the study/experiment.	
Collect the data.	
	Confirm and close the study (verify trustworthiness of the data).
	Interpret data in an ongoing manner throughout the study.
Disseminate the findings.	

REVIEW QUESTIONS

1. Which statement would the nurse manager evaluate as indicating a candidate for a position has information literacy?
   1. "I have a laptop and a smartphone I use regularly."
   2. "My last job required that I locate, evaluate, and use information on a daily basis."
   3. "My nursing school required that all papers be submitted electronically."
   4. "I use a word processing program to communicate with my family."

2. A nurse has appraised and synthesized a research article to help answer a clinical question. Which type of evidence is this nurse using?
   1. external
   2. clinical expertise
   3. internal
   4. patient preference

3. While evaluating a research study found online, the nurse identifies that the researcher included sparse information about the length of the study. Which part of the PICOT question is this nurse appraising?
   1. P
   2. I
   3. C
   4. T

4. The nurse is reviewing a journal article listed as including Level VII evidence. What should the nurse consider about this article?
   1. The article reflects meta-analyses of trials.
   2. The article reflects opinions of authorities or expert committees.
   3. Case-control or cohort studies were used to obtain data.
   4. The recommendations are based on systematic reviews of other studies.

5. A nurse determines that a study reported in an online source has no external validity. What does the nurse know about this study?
   1. The study intervention did not have a result on the outcome.
   2. This was a single-blind study.
   3. The results of the study are not generalizable.
   4. It is not clear that the dependent variable was influenced by the independent variable.

6. A nurse researcher is studying the effect of maternal caffeine intake on infant birth weight. Which type of variable is the amount of caffeine ingested?
   1. conceptual
   2. operational
   3. independent
   4. dependent

7. A researcher has this data: 3, 3, 3, 4, 4, 5, 6, 6, 7. Which of these is the mode?
   1. 3
   2. 5
   3. 3–7
   4. 4.56

Health and Illness Care of Adults

LEARNING OUTCOMES

1. Define health and discuss factors affecting the health of individuals, families, and communities.
2. Compare and contrast health risks, assessment, and health promotion for the young adult, middle adult, and older adult.
3. Discuss the nurse's role in health promotion.
4. Differentiate between disease and illness.
5. Describe illness behaviors and needs of the patient with acute illness and chronic illness.
6. Describe essential elements and goals of coordinated primary care models such as the Transitional Care Model and the Patient-Centered Medical Home.
7. Describe services, settings, and essential components of community-based care and home healthcare.
8. Discuss nursing interventions to deliver safe, effective, and competent care to patients in their homes.

CLINICAL COMPETENCIES

1. Use knowledge of individual and family variables to promote, restore, and maintain health when planning and implementing patient-centered care for adults.
2. Engage patients, family members, and other health team members in active partnerships to promote and maintain the health and safety of the adult.
3. Use high-quality electronic sources to plan and promote health for the adult.
4. Base individualized plans to promote and maintain health status on patient values, current evidence, and standards of practice.
5. Provide safe and effective individualized patient care in community-based settings and the home.
6. Use quality measures to evaluate and improve community-based and home care for adults.

TERMS MATCHING

Place the letter of the correct definition in the space next to each term.

1. _____ acute illness
2. _____ chronic illness
3. _____ community-based care
4. _____ disease
5. _____ exacerbation
6. _____ family
7. _____ health
8. _____ health–illness continuum
9. _____ holistic healthcare
10. _____ home healthcare
11. _____ hospice care
12. _____ illness
13. _____ manifestations
14. _____ patient-centered medical home (PCMH)
15. _____ primary care
16. _____ rehabilitation
17. _____ remission
18. _____ respite care
19. _____ transitional care
20. _____ wellness

A. A period of time during a chronic condition in which symptoms reappear

B. A period in which symptoms are not experienced even though the disease is still clinically present

C. An illness that occurs rapidly, lasts for a relatively short time, and is self-limiting

D. Signs and symptoms of a disease or condition caused by alterations in structure or function

E. Two or more persons joined by emotional closeness and shared bonds and who identify themselves as being part of a family

F. A state of complete physical, mental, and social well-being and not merely the absence of disease or infirmity

G. A visual representation of health as a dynamic process, with high-level wellness at one extreme and death at the opposite extreme

H. The response a person has to a disease; integrates the patient's perception, as well as the pathophysiologic alterations and the psychologic effects of those alterations

I. A condition that requires continuing management over a long period—years or even decades

J. A philosophy of healthcare in which all aspects of a person (physical, psychosocial, cultural, spiritual, and intellectual) are considered as essential components of individualized care

K. A medical term describing alterations in structure and function of the body or mind that may have mechanical, biologic, or normative causes

L. Provides short-term or intermittent home care, often using volunteers

M. An integrated method of functioning oriented toward maximizing an individual's potential within the environment

N. The delivery of services to restore or maintain the health of individuals and families in the home

O. Accessible, comprehensive, and coordinated primary care focused on illness prevention for patients and families

P. Centers on individual and family healthcare needs; care provided in the local community that is culturally competent and family centered

Q. Comprehensive first-contact health and illness care across the life span

R. Interventions designed to improve the ability of patients and caregivers to manage care needs in preparation for transitions from one healthcare setting to another or to home

S. Special component of home care, designed to provide medical, nursing, social, psychologic, and spiritual care for terminally ill patients and their families

T. The process of learning to live to one's maximum potential with a chronic impairment and its resultant functional disability

FOCUSED STUDY

1. List and describe factors that affect health.

a.

_____

b.

_____

c.

_____

d.

_____

e.

_____

f.

_____

g.

_____

h.

_____

2. Identify the generally accepted common causes of disease.

a.

_____

b.

_____

c.

_____

d.

_____

e.

_____

f.

_____

g.

3. Describe the difference between acute and chronic illness.

_____

_____

_____

_____

4. Define and give examples of primary, secondary, and tertiary illness prevention activities.

a. Primary activities:

_____

_____

b. Secondary activities:

_____

_____

c. Tertiary activities:

_____

CASE STUDY

Jacob is a 50-year-old African American unemployed male with a history of past substance abuse who is being counseled about health promotion activities. Answer the following questions based on your knowledge of the middle-aged adult and Jacob's history.

1. What alterations in health is Jacob at risk for developing as a middle-aged adult?

2. What psychosocial stressors are likely for Jacob?

3. How can the nurse promote healthy behaviors in Jacob?

SHORT ANSWERS

Fill in the information table for recommended adult immunizations.

Vaccine	Indications	Do not give to
Measles-mumps-rubella		Pregnant women, immunocompromised people, or anyone with a history of anaphylactic reaction to egg protein or neomycin.
Tetanus, diptheria, pertussis (Td, Tdap)	All adults should receive 1 dose of Tdap followed by a Td booster every 10 years.	
Hepatitis A		
Hepatitis B		People with a history of anaphylactic reaction to common baker's yeast.
Human papillomavirus (HPV)		People with a history of anaphylactic reaction to the vaccine or its components.
Influenza	All adults should receive annual immunization against seasonal influenza.	
Meningococcal disease		People with a severe allergic reaction to vaccine component or following a prior dose of vaccine; those currently experiencing moderate or severe acute illness.
Pneumococcal pneumonia	Anyone at high risk for pneumococcal disease and those _____ of age.	
Varicella		Pregnant women, immunocompromised people, those who _____ within 5 months, or those with a history of anaphylactic reactions to neomycin or gelatin.
Zoster (shingles)		Pregnant women, immunocompromised people, and those with a history of anaphylactic reactions to neomycin or gelatin.

REVIEW QUESTIONS

1. Identify the acute illness from the following illnesses.
   1. influenza
   2. cancer
   3. hemophilia
   4. sickle cell disease
2. Which relationship is an example of an altered response of health to lifestyle and environmental influences?
   1. cigarette smoking to a sedentary lifestyle
   2. alcoholism to obesity
   3. obesity to hypertension
   4. a sedentary lifestyle to chronic obstructive pulmonary disease

3. Which practice is not known to promote health and wellness?
   1. sleeping 5–6 hours each day
   2. smoking cessation
   3. keeping sun exposure to a minimum
   4. maintaining recommended immunizations

4. The patient demonstrates behaviors of self-preoccupation during the initial assessment. This behavior is characteristic of what stage of illness?
   1. experiencing symptoms
   2. assuming a dependent role
   3. achieving recovery and rehabilitation
   4. assuming the sick role

5. Given that the patient is 35 years old, the nurse knows that the patient would fall into which stage of adulthood?
   1. young adult
   2. middle adult
   3. older adult
   4. young middle adult

6. Identify the cancer not commonly found in the middle adult.
   1. lung
   2. liver
   3. reproductive
   4. colon

7. Which condition does not frequently occur in the older adult?
   1. hypertension
   2. arthritis
   3. sinusitis
   4. obesity

8. Identify the ineffective coping skill of a patient with a chronic illness.
   1. learning to adapt activities of daily living and self-care activities
   2. denying the inevitability of death
   3. complying with a medical treatment plan
   4. maintaining a feeling of being in control

CHAPTER 4

Nursing Care of Patients Having Surgery

LEARNING OUTCOMES

1. Compare the differences and similarities between outpatient and inpatient surgery.
2. Identify the three phases of perioperative care.
3. Interpret the significance of data used in the perioperative period to determine the patient's health status and risk profile.
4. Explain nursing implications for medications prescribed for the surgical patient.
5. Identify variations in perioperative care for patients across the life span and with differing needs based on culture.
6. Describe principles of pain management specific to acute postoperative pain control.
7. Differentiate the care needed for patients receiving varying levels of anesthesia care.

CLINICAL COMPETENCIES

1. Assess the physiologic and psychosocial health status of patients scheduled for surgery to determine their ability to tolerate surgery and identify risks for complications.
2. Develop an understanding of patient-centered care based on a respect for patient's preference, values, and needs prior to anesthesia, during postoperative care, and prior to discharge from the facility.
3. Function effectively within an interprofessional team using written and oral techniques to minimize risks associated with handoffs among team members during transitions between phases of the perioperative experience.
4. Observe and participate as appropriate with nursing responsibilities and interventions that integrate best current evidence to promote quality and patient safety in the perioperative environment.
5. Use the nursing process and technology to plan, provide, and document safe and effective nursing care for the patient in the preoperative, intraoperative, and postoperative phases of surgery.

TERMS MATCHING

Place the letter of the correct definition in the space next to each term.

1. _____ anesthesia
2. _____ anesthesia care provider (ACP)
3. _____ circulating nurse
4. _____ conscious sedation
5. _____ dehiscence
6. _____ evisceration
7. _____ general anesthesia
8. _____ handoff
9. _____ informed consent
10. _____ intraoperative phase
11. _____ perioperative nursing
12. _____ postoperative phase
13. _____ preoperative phase
14. _____ regional anesthesia
15. _____ scrub person
16. _____ surgery

A. The disclosure of risks associated with the intended procedure or operation to the patient. The language of the document varies according to statutory and common law of each state

B. A type of anesthesia providing analgesia, amnesia, and moderate sedation, allowing the patient to respond to verbal and physical stimulation

C. Time when preparation of the patient for surgery is conducted and completed

D. Healthcare professional who has responsibility for providing anesthesia during the operative experience

E. An unintended separation of wound margins due to incomplete healing

F. An experienced registered nurse who coordinates and manages a wide range of activities before, during, and after a surgical procedure; the duties include overseeing the physical aspects of the operating room and equipment, assisting with the transfer and positioning of the patient, preparing the patient's skin, ensuring that no break in aseptic technique occurs, and counting all sponges and instruments

G. Protrusion of body contents through a surgical wound

H. A specialized area of nursing practice incorporating the three phases of the surgical experience: preoperative, intraoperative, and postoperative

I. The time during surgery, from beginning to end

J. Period when a procedure or surgery has been completed and the patient is recovering from the stress associated with the surgery

K. Prepares the sterile field, surgical supplies, and equipment for surgical procedures; also assists surgeon and physician assistant by passing instruments, suctioning blood, and maintaining the sterile field

L. Use of drugs to produce sedation, analgesia, reflex loss, and muscle relaxation during a surgical procedure

M. An invasive medical procedure performed to diagnose or treat illness, injury, or deformity

N. Anesthesia that desensitizes the area to be operated but does not involve the full central nervous system or cause sedation

O. Deep sedation, which includes analgesia and muscle paralysis. This type of anesthesia requires respiratory maintenance without the aid of the patient's respiratory musculature.

P. Procedure whereby responsibility for patient care is transferred from one individual or care unit to another

FOCUSED STUDY

1. List and describe the three phases of the perioperative experience.

a.

_____

b.

_____

c.

_____

2. Describe the role and responsibilities of the following healthcare providers within the perioperative setting.

a. Surgeon

_____

b. Circulating nurse

_____

c. Scrub person

_____

d. Anesthesiologist or CRNA

_____

e. Phlebotomist

_____

f. X-ray technician

_____

g. Transporter

_____

3. Describe the differences between general anesthesia, regional anesthesia, and conscious sedation.

_____

_____

_____

_____

_____

4. Describe the following postoperative complications and their appropriate nursing interventions.

a. Hemorrhage:

_____

_____

_____

b. Deep vein thrombosis:

_____

_____

_____

c. Pneumonia:

_____

_____

_____

CASE STUDY

Mrs. Elvira, a 28-year-old female, is scheduled to undergo a right radical mastectomy. Mrs. Elvira reports smoking two-and-a-half packs of cigarettes a day and obtaining minimal exercise. She takes aspirin for frequent headaches and herbal supplements to help her lose weight. Answer the following questions based on your knowledge of patient needs for undergoing surgery.

1. Mrs. Elvira's informed consent document includes the surgeon's name, the alternatives and risks of treatments, and the date and time she and her surgeon signed the consent. What is missing?

2. What postoperative complication(s) is Mrs. Elvira at most risk of developing based on her history?

3. What preoperative studies and interventions will Mrs. Elvira undergo to reduce the likelihood of intraoperative and postoperative complications?

4. Prior to discharge, Mrs. Elvira will be instructed to assess her incision site for signs of infection. What are they?

SHORT ANSWERS

1. Complete the following chart.

Classification of Medication	Potential Surgical Complication	Nursing Care
Anticoagulants/platelet inhibitors		
Antidepressants (particularly monoamine oxidase inhibitors)		
Antihypertensives		
Antibiotics (particularly the "mycin" group)		
Diuretics		
Herbal supplements		
Immunosuppressants		

REVIEW QUESTIONS

1. Informed consent must include which information? **Select all that apply.**
   1. description and purpose of the proposed procedure
   2. alternative treatments or procedures available
   3. date, time, and location of the proposed surgical procedure
   4. right to refuse treatment or withdraw consent
   5. potential complications
2. The nurse is working to orient a new nurse in the postanesthesia care unit. Which of the following actions by the new nurse indicates an understanding of methods to prevent hypothermia?
   1. The nurse monitors the patient's temperature every 15 minutes.
   2. The nurse monitors the patient's blood pressure every 30 minutes.
   3. Upon the patient's arrival in postanesthesia care unit and after sterile drapes are removed, the nurse applies warm blankets.
   4. The nurse advises the patient to report feelings of coldness.
3. After the patient has undergone surgery with a spinal anesthetic, she develops a postoperative spinal headache. Which intervention is appropriate for the nurse to implement?
   1. Decrease patient hydration.
   2. Raise the head of the bed 45 degrees.
   3. Prepare the patient for a blood patch procedure.
   4. Restrict all caffeine products.

4. Identify the surgical team member who is responsible for documenting intraoperative nursing activities, medications, blood administration, placement of drains and catheters, and length of the procedure.
   1. surgeon
   2. circulating nurse
   3. Certified Registered Nurse Anesthetist
   4. surgical scrub

5. What is an outcome of improper intraoperative surgical positioning?
   1. nerve damage
   2. hyperthermia
   3. hemorrhage
   4. increased joint flexibility

6. The nurse knows that the patient understood perioperative teaching when the patient demonstrates which of these behaviors?
   1. arrives with freshly painted nails
   2. has eaten a full breakfast before arriving at the hospital
   3. has completed all preoperative testing as ordered
   4. arrives with contacts in place

7. The patient has a positive Homans' sign after surgery. Which intervention, planned by a nursing student, indicates the need for further education?
   1. assessing the extremity for redness
   2. asking the preceptor about discontinuing the patient's anticoagulant
   3. recording bilateral calf or thigh circumferences every shift
   4. teaching and supporting the patient and family

8. Which assessment finding is uncommon in a patient who is experiencing symptoms of a pulmonary embolism?
   1. anxiety
   2. decreased oxygen saturation
   3. decrease in respiratory rate
   4. cough

Nursing Care of Patients Experiencing Loss, Grief, and Death

LEARNING OUTCOMES

1. Explain how theories of loss and grief influence provision of patient-centered care for individuals experiencing loss, grief, and death.
2. Explain factors affecting patient and family responses to loss.
3. Analyze common legal and ethical issues in end-of-life care.
4. Describe the philosophy and activities of hospice and palliative care.
5. Describe the physiologic responses associated with the end of life.

CLINICAL COMPETENCIES

1. Recognize physiologic changes in the dying patient.
2. Use assessments, patient values, and evidence-based practice guidelines to provide nursing interventions that enhance quality of life and promote a comfortable and dignified death for patients and their families.
3. Use principles of palliative care to manage pain and other symptoms associated with the end of life.
4. Effectively communicate with and function within the interprofessional team to plan and provide individualized care for patients and families experiencing loss, grief, and death.
5. Integrate individual and cultural values and variations, as well as expressed needs and preferences, into the plan of care for patients and families experiencing loss, grief, and death.
6. Identify self-care strategies to use when caring for patients and families experiencing loss, grief, and death.

TERMS MATCHING

Place the letter of the correct definition in the space next to each term.

1. _____ advance directive
2. _____ aid in dying
3. _____ assisted suicide
4. _____ bereavement
5. _____ chronic sorrow
6. _____ death
7. _____ death anxiety
8. _____ delirium
9. _____ do-not-resuscitate order
10. _____ durable power of attorney
11. _____ end-of-life
12. _____ euthanasia
13. _____ grief
14. _____ grieving
15. _____ healthcare surrogate
16. _____ hospice
17. _____ living will
18. _____ loss
19. _____ mourning
20. _____ palliative care
21. _____ physician orders for life-sustaining treatment (POLST)

A. An irreversible cessation of circulatory and respiratory functions or irreversible cessation of all functions of the entire brain, including the brainstem

B. From the Greek for painless, easy, gentle, or good death, now commonly used to signify a killing prompted by some humanitarian motive

C. The final days or weeks of life when death is imminent

D. A special component of home care, designed to provide medical, nursing, social, psychologic, and spiritual care for terminally ill patients and their families

E. Actions or expressions of the bereaved

F. Care focused on the relief of physical, mental, and spiritual distress for individuals who have an incurable illness

G. The means to end a patient's life is provided to the patient with knowledge of the patient's intention

H. The emotional response to loss and its accompanying changes

I. An individual selected to make medical decisions when another person can no longer make them

J. An actual or potential situation in which a valued object, person, body part, or emotion that was formerly present is lost or changed and can no longer be seen, felt, heard, known, or experienced

K. Worry or fear related to death or dying

L. A document that can delegate the authority to make health, financial, and/or legal decisions on a person's behalf

M. A document that provides written directions about life-prolonging procedures to provide instructions when a person can no longer communicate in a life-threatening situation

N. The time of mourning experienced after a loss

O. Usually written by the physician for the patient who has a terminal illness or is near death, this order is usually based on the wishes of the patient and family that no cardiopulmonary resuscitation be performed for respiratory or cardiac arrest

P. The internal process the person uses to work through the response to loss

Q. A cyclical, recurring, and potentially progressive pattern of pervasive sadness experienced in response to continual loss, throughout the trajectory of an illness or disability

R. An end-of-life care option in which mentally competent, terminally ill adults ask their physician to provide a prescription for medication that the patient can self-administer to end life peacefully

S. Also called a *living will*, this is a document in which a patient formally states preferences for healthcare in the event that he or she later becomes mentally incapacitated, and names a person who has durable power of attorney to serve as a substitute decision maker to implement the patient's stated preferences

T. A state of consciousness when the patient may be restless, confused, or agitated

U. A form for patients with serious, progressive, chronic illnesses that translates their wishes regarding life-sustaining treatment into actionable medical orders

FOCUSED STUDY

1. Describe the philosophy and activities of hospice and palliative care.

_____

_____

_____

_____

_____

2. List the manifestations of impending death.

_____

_____

_____

_____

3. Cultural care is as important at the end of life as it is at any other time during the patient's life. Discuss nursing interventions with regard to the cultural considerations of a variety of ethnic groups regarding end-of-life care.

_____

_____

_____

_____

_____

_____

CASE STUDY

You are the hospice nurse for 27-year-old Alana Oberan. She recently received a terminal diagnosis of an aggressive form of cancer and has been informed by her physician that a 4-month survival rate would be optimistic. Alana's support system consists of both of her parents. Answer the following questions based on your knowledge of grief and end-of-life care.

1. Discuss spiritual assessment, including questions to consider during this assessment process.

2. Discuss Kübler-Ross's stages of death and dying, including reactions that may occur during the grieving process.

3. What factors will affect the parents' ability to grieve their upcoming loss?

CROSSWORD PUZZLE

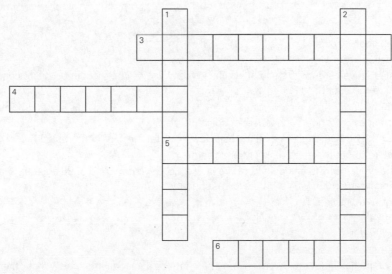

Across

3   A killing prompted by some humanitarian motive
4   Stage of grief in which the person's behavior becomes disorganized
5   A combination of intellectual and emotional responses and behaviors by which people adjust their self-concept in the face of an actual or potential loss
6   Kübler-Ross stage of grief in which individual resists loss

Down

1   A healthcare _____ is an individual selected to make medical decisions when another person is no longer able to do so
2   Legal document that allows a person to plan for healthcare by providing written directions about life prolonging procedures

REVIEW QUESTIONS

1. After the physician leaves the room, the nurse enters and finds the patient crying. What would be the best statement for the nurse to make to the patient?
   1. "The physician said that she told you about your testing tomorrow. Is that true?"
   2. "Is there someone I can call for you?"
   3. "Tell me what concerns you the most."
   4. "Are you upset about tomorrow's testing?"

2. After providing care for a dying patient, the nurse documents the care. What is the best evaluation statement in regard to the grieving process?
   1. Oral care provided, patient repositioned for comfort
   2. Mucous membranes moist and intact
   3. Oxygen applied via nasal cannula
   4. Patient confused, sister at bedside

3. A patient is unresponsive after 6 months of aggressive treatment for pancreatic cancer. What document would allow a designated person to make decisions about the patient's healthcare?
   1. advanced directive
   2. durable power of attorney
   3. living will
   4. Patient's Bill of Rights

4. The patient has a do-not-resuscitate order on the chart, and the family has decided to provide palliative care rather than aggressive treatment. What nursing intervention is an appropriate nursing response to the patient's moans and grimaces?
   1. Administer 2 mg IV morphine per the physician's order.
   2. Assess for pain, reposition the patient, and then reassess for pain.
   3. Ask the family if this is how the patient reacts to pain.
   4. Call the physician to seek a long-term pain control medication.

5. A patient asks the nurse about the reputation of the physician who diagnosed his colon cancer. The patient states, "I should get another opinion before I have this surgery tomorrow." In which stage of grief is this patient? **Select all that apply**.
   1. Kübler-Ross: anger
   2. Engel: restitution
   3. Bowlby: protest
   4. Lindemann: morbid grief reaction
   5. Caplan: stress and loss

6. The patient chooses palliative care for the end of his life. What would be the most appropriate action for the nurse to take in the last hours of the patient's life?
   1. Take vital signs hourly.
   2. Reposition the patient every 2 hours if needed for comfort.
   3. Elevate the head of the bed 90 degrees at all times and administer 4 mg of IV morphine.
   4. Encourage the patient to eat to keep up his or her strength.

7. The patient at the end of life reports being short of breath with a respiratory rate of 38 and an oxygen saturation of 92%. Which nursing intervention would be the lowest priority?
   1. Administer 2 mg of IV morphine.
   2. Administer oxygen 2 L/min via nasal cannula.
   3. Elevate the head of bed.
   4. Gently suction the patient's nasopharynx.

8. A patient at the end of life has intractable vomiting and has refused a nasogastric tube. What other nursing interventions may aid the patient's comfort?
   1. Encourage the patient to drink ginger ale with ice chips.
   2. Administer morphine 1 mg IV.
   3. Administer prochlorperazine (Compazine) PO.
   4. Administer ondansetron (Zofran) IV.

Nursing Care of Patients with **Problems** of **Substance Abuse**

LEARNING OUTCOMES

1. Recognize the pathophysiology, manifestations, and complications of substance abuse.
2. Discuss risk factors associated with substance abuse.
3. Describe common characteristics of people with substance abuse problems.
4. Explain the effects of addictive substances on physiological, cognitive, psychologic, and social well-being.
5. Support interprofessional care for the patient with substance abuse problems, including diagnostic tests, emergency care for overdose, and treatment of withdrawal.
6. Recognize the potential for substance abuse in coworkers.

CLINICAL COMPETENCIES

1. Assess and monitor the health status of patients with substance abuse or dependence.
2. Monitor for signs of withdrawal and life-threatening conditions.
3. Provide skilled nursing care during the detoxification period, respecting expressed needs, values, and preferences.
4. Collaborate and coordinate with the patient and other members of the interprofessional team when caring for patients with substance abuse problems.
5. Educate patients about stress management, coping skills, nutrition, relapse prevention, and healthy lifestyle choices.
6. Using assessed data and current standards of practice, plan and implement individualized nursing care for patients experiencing problems with substance abuse.
7. Evaluate patient responses to care, revising the plan of care as needed to promote, maintain, or restore functional health status to patients with substance abuse problems.
8. Participate in studies and projects to improve outcomes for patients with substance abuse disorders.
9. Apply technology and information management tools to support safe processes of care for patients with substance abuse disorders.

TERMS MATCHING

Place the letter of the correct definition in the space next to each term.

1. _____ alcohol
2. _____ amphetamine
3. _____ caffeine
4. _____ cannabis sativa
5. _____ central nervous system depressants
6. _____ cocaine
7. _____ co-occurring disorders
8. _____ delirium tremens (DT)
9. _____ hallucinogens
10. _____ inhalants
11. _____ Korsakoff's psychosis
12. _____ nicotine
13. _____ opiates
14. _____ polysubstance abuse
15. _____ psychostimulants
16. _____ substance abuse
17. _____ substance dependence
18. _____ tolerance
19. _____ Wernicke's encephalopathy
20. _____ withdrawal
21. _____ withdrawal symptoms

A. A cumulative state in which a particular dose of a chemical elicits a smaller response than before

B. Drugs that produce hallucinations, also referred to as psychedelics, including phencyclidine (PCP), 3,4-methylenedioxy-methamphetamine (MDMA), d-lysergic acid diethylamide (LSD), mescaline, dimethyltryptamine (DMT), and psilocin

C. A medical emergency that usually occurs 2–5 days following alcohol withdrawal and persists for 2–3 days

D. The use of any chemical in a fashion inconsistent with medical or culturally defined social norms despite physical, psychologic, or social adverse effects

E. Analgesics derived from the opium plant; produce analgesia by binding to opioid receptors within and outside the CNS; the most potent analgesics available, and the treatment of choice for acute moderate-to-severe pain

F. Inhaled solvents categorized into three types: anesthetics, volatile nitrites, and organic solvents

G. A stimulant found in tobacco that enters the system via the lungs (cigarettes and cigars) and oral mucous membranes (chewing tobacco as well as smoking)

H. A central nervous system depressant that is the most commonly abused drug

I. Highly addictive substances such as cocaine and amphetamines that give the user a sense of euphoria

J. Concurrent diagnosis of a substance-use disorder and a psychiatric disorder

K. The source of marijuana

L. The simultaneous use of many substances

M. A severe condition occurring when the use of a chemical substance is no longer under an individual's control for at least 3 months

N. A condition seen in chronic alcoholism as a result of thiamine (B_1) deficiency that is characterized by nystagmus, ptosis, ataxia, confusion, coma, and possible death

O. A constellation of signs and symptoms that occurs in physically dependent individuals when they discontinue the use of a substance

P. A methylxanthine stimulant found in soft drinks, coffee, tea, chocolate, and some pain relievers that increases the heart rate and acts as a diuretic

Q. A stimulant that causes arousal and mood elevation with decreased need for food or sleep but increased risk for mental disorders

R. Secondary dementia caused by thiamine (B1) deficiency that may be associated with chronic alcoholism; characterized by progressive cognitive deterioration, confabulation, peripheral neuropathy, and myopathy

S. Cessation of use of a substance to which an individual has become addicted

T. A highly addictive stimulant/euphoric drug extracted from the leaves of the coca plant

U. Substances such as barbiturates, benzodiazepines, paraldehyde, meprobamate, and chloral hydrate, which are subject to abuse

FOCUSED STUDY

1. Explain the following risk factors as they relate to substance abuse.
   a. Genetic factors

   _____

   _____

   b. Biologic factors

   _____

   _____

   c. Psychologic factors

   _____

   _____

   d. Sociocultural factors

   _____

   _____

2. Complete the following table.

Addictive Substance	Effect
Caffeine	
Nicotine	
Cannabis	
Alcohol	
CNS depressants	
Psychostimulants	
Amphetamines	
Opiates	
Hallucinogens	
Inhalants	

3. Describe the following substance abuse screening tools.
   a. Michigan Alcohol Screening Test (MAST) brief version

   _____

   _____

   b. CAGE questionnaire

   _____

   _____

   c. Brief Drug Abuse Screening Test (B-DAST)

   _____

   _____

4. Identify community-based care options available to patients who suffer from substance abuse.

   _____

   _____

   _____

   _____

CASE STUDY

Ryan Dern is a 32-year-old male who suffers from alcoholism. He has taken the initial step of admitting to his problem and seeking medical assistance. Answer the following questions based on your knowledge of alcoholism.

1. How long does Ryan need to have had excessive drinking behaviors to be considered substance-dependent?

2. What factors affect the rate of alcohol absorption?

3. What vitamin deficiency is associated with alcoholism? How will the nurse assist Ryan in meeting his nutritional needs?

4. The nurse will teach Ryan HALT. What is HALT?

CROSSWORD PUZZLE

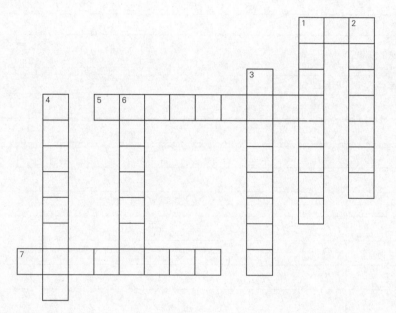

Across

1 The psychoactive component of marijuana
5 Substance derived from cannabis sativa that is the most commonly abused illegal drug in the United States
7 Long-term changes in brain neurotransmission that occur after repeated detoxifications

Down

1 Vitamin deficiency commonly seen in alcoholics
2 Street term commonly used to refer to methamphetamine
3 Stimulant found in food and beverages that increases heart rate
4 The primary subjective effect associated with cocaine and amphetamines
6 Most commonly abused legal drug in the United States

REVIEW QUESTIONS

1. Identify the neurotransmitter that plays a pivotal role in substance abuse.
1. dopamine
2. endorphin
3. enkephalin
4. dynorphin

2. Which ethnic group reports the lowest incidence of alcohol abuse?
1. African Americans
2. Native Americans
3. Hispanics
4. Asians

3. Which addictive substance may be a risk factor in developing future psychotic symptoms?
1. cocaine
2. methamphetamine
3. cannabis
4. OxyContin®

4. The patient reports to the nurse that he has been using crank. The nurse knows that crank is a form of what substance?
1. methamphetamine
2. opiate
3. hallucinogen
4. alcohol

5. Which body fluids are often tested for drug content? **Select all that apply**.
1. saliva
2. tears
3. urine
4. blood
5. stool

6. Which is the correct form of questioning to use when assessing a patient for substance abuse?
1. "You don't have any drug abusers in your family, do you?"
2. "Did you ever abuse a substance in the past?"
3. "Have you ever been treated in an alcohol or drug abuse clinic?"
4. "Were you ever arrested for a driving while under the influence (DUI) offense?"

7. Which screening tool is most effective for the nurse to use when the patient does not recognize his or her substance abuse problem?
1. Brief Drug Abuse Screening Test (B-DAST)
2. CAGE questionnaire
3. Michigan Alcohol Screening Test (MAST) brief version
4. HALT Screening Assessment tool

8. The nurse caring for a patient with a substance abuse addiction should employ which intervention?
1. Assess the patient's level of disorientation.
2. Place the patient alone in a private room.
3. Accept the use of defense mechanisms.
4. Do not encourage the patient to verbalize anxieties.

9. Nurses have a higher incidence of what type of substance abuse?
1. alcohol
2. hallucinogen
3. opiate
4. amphetamine

CHAPTER 7

Nursing Care of Patients Experiencing Disasters

LEARNING OUTCOMES

1. Explain the difference between an emergency and a disaster.
2. Describe the types of injuries and manifestations associated with biologic, chemical, or radiologic terrorism.
3. Describe accepted triage principles used to manage multiple or mass casualty incidents and disasters.
4. Recognize situations requiring the need for patient isolation or patient decontamination.
5. Discuss the role of the nurse in disaster preparedness, mitigation, response, and recovery.
6. Discuss common nursing interventions for the treatment of injuries related to biologic, chemical, or radiologic terrorism.
7. Identify federal, state, local, and voluntary resources that provide support and assistance with disaster preparedness, response, and recovery.

CLINICAL COMPETENCIES

1. Activate a personal and family disaster plan to allow for your participation in disaster response.
2. Apply accepted triage tools and systems adopted by local emergency medical services and hospitals to establish care based on disaster situation and available resources.
3. Adapt evidence-based standards of nursing practice, based on resources available, to implement nursing care for patients with injuries suffered as a result of a disaster.
4. Provide safe and knowledgeable nursing care to treat disaster-related injuries.
5. Evaluate and revise the plan of care to restore functional health status to patients who have sustained injuries due to a disaster.
6. Maintain personal safety and the safety of others at the scene of a disaster.
7. Provide education to promote participation in core preparedness activities.

TERMS MATCHING

Place the letter of the correct definition in the space next to each term.

1. _____ bioterrorism
2. _____ cold zone
3. _____ conventional weapons
4. _____ disasters
5. _____ emergency
6. _____ evaluation phase
7. _____ hot zone
8. _____ human-generated disasters
9. _____ mass casualty incidents (MCIs)
10. _____ mitigation
11. _____ natural disasters
12. _____ nonconventional terrorist weapons
13. _____ personal protective equipment (PPE)
14. _____ preparedness
15. _____ radiation sickness
16. _____ recovery
17. _____ response
18. _____ reverse triage
19. _____ surge capacity
20. _____ terrorism
21. _____ triage
22. _____ warm zone

A. Complex emergencies, technologic situations, material shortages, and other situations that are produced by identifiable human actions, deliberate or otherwise

B. Actions that address preparations for and actions in dealing with the consequences of a disaster

C. An unforeseen combination of circumstances that calls for immediate action for a range of victims from one to many

D. A healthcare system's ability to rapidly expand beyond normal services to meet the increased demand for qualified personnel, medical care, and public health in the event of a large-scale disaster

E. During a mass casualty event, victims who are most severely injured, requiring extensive resources with little chance of surviving, are treated last

F. The site of the disaster where a weapon was released or where the contamination occurred

G. The fifth of 5 stages of disaster. Activities include rebuilding and returning to some semblance of "normalcy" but also include mitigation activities or planning to prevent subsequent disasters or to minimize the effects of future disasters

H. Natural or human-generated events that require extraordinary efforts beyond those needed to respond to everyday emergencies

I. These are produced by acts of nature or emerging diseases; they may be predictable through advanced meteorologic technologies or they may be unexpected

J. The action taken to prevent or reduce the harmful effects of a disaster on human health or property; involves future-oriented activities to prevent subsequent disasters or to minimize their effects

K. Equipment used for the protection of personnel; includes gloves, masks, goggles, gowns, and biologic disposal bags

L. One of the results of DNA mutation inside cells exposed to ionizing radiation.

M. All types of bombs and guns

N. The U.S. Department of Defense defines this term as the "calculated use of violence or the threat of violence to inculcate fear; intended to coerce or to intimidate governments or societies in the pursuit of goals that are generally political, religious or ideological"

O. Situations in which 100 or more casualties are involved, significantly overwhelming available emergency medical services, facilities, and resources

P. Use of etiologic agents (disease) with deliberate intent to cause harm or kill or death in a population, food, and/or livestock

Q. This is a safe area next to the warm zone and where in-depth triage of victims can occur; survivors may find shelter in this area, and the command and control vehicles would be located here as well

R. Chemicals, biologic agents, and nuclear agents used to harm or kill a population

S. This area is adjacent to the hot zone and is also referred to as the *control zone*; this is where decontamination of victims or triage and emergency treatment can occur

T. The final phase of disaster planning that involves a detailed review of a disaster relief program to determine if goals were met, to assess the program's impact on the community and to identify lessons learned for the design of future plans

U. Means "sorting"; a continuous process in which patient priorities are reassigned as needed treatments, time, and the condition of the patients change

V. Phase occurring immediately after the impact of the disaster event has occurred

FOCUSED STUDY

1. Describe the differences between an emergency and a disaster. Provide one example of each.

_____

_____

_____

_____

2. Provide examples of conventional weapons and nonconventional terrorist weapons.

_____

_____

_____

_____

_____

3. Describe the difference between triage and reverse triage. Provide an example of when each system should be utilized.

_____

_____

_____

_____

_____

CASE STUDY

Mrs. Deckman, a 72-year-old female, has been trapped in her home as a result of a hurricane and flooding. She is a diabetic who controls her blood sugar with oral hypoglycemics. She has no other significant past medical history. Answer the following questions based on your knowledge of the care of patients experiencing disasters.

1. What is a hurricane?

2. What physical effects of a hurricane is Mrs. Deckman at risk for, regardless of her past medical history?

3. Mrs. Deckman was classified with a triage level of "red" after she was taken to a local shelter. What does this mean?

4. Mrs. Deckman asks the nurse for assistance in developing a disaster box to be used in case of another disaster. What items should the nurse suggest to be kept in the box?

5. What is the role of the nurse who works with the victims of this natural disaster?

6. A crowd has developed at the site of the shelter where Mrs. Deckman is being treated. What is one consequence of poor crowd management?

SHORT ANSWERS

List types of injuries that may be seen in victims of chemical and radiologic terrorism. Briefly describe three nursing interventions that should be provided for these two types of terrorism.

Type of Terrorism	Chemical	Radiologic
Types of injuries	1.	1.
	2.	2.
Nursing interventions	1.	1.
	2.	2.
	3.	3.

REVIEW QUESTIONS

1. Identify the nonconventional terrorist weapon.
   1. incendiary bomb
   2. shoulder-fired missiles
   3. anthrax
   4. hand grenade

2. Which items are sources of ionizing radiation? **Select all that apply.**
   1. stars
   2. sun
   3. x-ray machines
   4. cell phones
   5. fire

3. The mitigation phase involves which types of activities?
   1. planning and preparation
   2. warning, preimpact mobilization, and evacuation
   3. the community experiencing the immediate effects
   4. the immediate response to the effects of the disaster

4. The nurse classifies a patient as "yellow" during the triage process. The yellow code identifies the patient as having which characteristic?
   1. requiring the most support and immediate emergency care
   2. being in less critical condition but still in need of transport to an emergency care center
   3. having only minor injuries, which does not warrant the victim's transport to an emergency center
   4. being least likely to survive or already deceased

5. Which term refers to the area where a weapon was released or where the contamination has occurred?
   1. cold zone
   2. warm zone
   3. hot zone
   4. danger zone

6. Overexertion and exhaustion are most often associated with which type of disasters?
   1. blast
   2. snow
   3. earthquake
   4. tornado

CHAPTER 8

Genetic Implications of Adult Health Nursing

LEARNING OUTCOMES

1. Discuss the role of genetic concepts in health promotion and health maintenance.
2. Apply knowledge of the principles of genetic transmission and risk factors for genetic disorders.
3. Describe the significance of delivering genetic education and counseling follow-up in a professional manner.
4. Explain the implications of genetic advances on the role of nurses, with particular attention to spiritual, cultural, ethical, legal, and social issues.
5. Identify the significance of recent advances in human genetics and the effect on healthcare delivery.

CLINICAL COMPETENCIES

1. Integrate genetic assessment and the use of a pedigree family history into delivery of nursing care.
2. Identify patients or families with actual or potential genetic conditions and initiate referrals to a genetics professional.
3. Prepare patients and their families for a genetic evaluation and facilitate the genetic counseling process.
4. Integrate basic genetic concepts into patient and family education with consideration of cultural and personal preferences and values of the family and the reinforcement of information provided to patients by genetic professionals.

TERMS MATCHING

Place the letter of the correct definition in the space next to each item.

1. _____ alleles
2. _____ autosomal dominant
3. _____ autosomal recessive
4. _____ autosomes
5. _____ biologic markers
6. _____ chromosomes
7. _____ gene
8. _____ genotype
9. _____ heterozygous
10. _____ homozygous
11. _____ human genome
12. _____ meiosis
13. _____ mitosis
14. _____ penetrance
15. _____ phenotype
16. _____ polymorphisms
17. _____ sex chromosomes
18. _____ somatic cell
19. _____ translocation
20. _____ trisomy 21
21. _____ X-linked recessive

A. The process of making new cells by cell division; results in two cells called daughter cells that are genetically identical to the original cell, or mother cell, and to each other

B. The genes and the variations therein that a person inherits from his or her parents

C. Nonidentical copies of a particular gene (different alleles) on the paired chromosomes

D. The reduction division of the cell occurring only in the sex cells of the testes and ovaries when the amount of genetic material is reduced in half (23 chromosomes)

E. The percentage or likelihood that an individual who has inherited a gene mutation will actually express the disease signs and symptoms in his or her lifetime

F. Different forms of a gene or DNA occupying the same place on a pair of chromosomes

G. Genetic conditions that result from an altered gene on any of the 22 autosomes in spite of the fact that one unaltered or normal gene exists

H. The observable, outward expression of an individual's entire physical, biochemical, and physiological makeup as determined by his or her genotype (alleles) and by environmental factors

I. The chromosomes X or Y that indicate gender

J. The result of an altered gene on the X chromosome. All males with this alteration will express the consequences due to only having one X chromosome. Females may not express the consequence if they have a second normal X chromosome

K. A single chromosome from any one of the 22 pairs of chromosomes not involved in sex determination (X or Y); humans have 22 pairs of these

L. Identical copies of a particular gene (same alleles) on both paired chromosomes

M. Any cell in the body that is not a sex cell (ova and sperm)

N. Stable segments of DNA

O. A sequence of DNA on a chromosome that represents a fundamental unit of heredity; occupies a specific spot on a chromosome (gene locus)

P. Genetic conditions that require two copies of an altered gene on any of the 22 autosomes to express the condition

Q. Down syndrome; an additional copy of chromosome 21 is present

R. Genetic material carried by each cell; found in the cell nucleus

S. The total amount of the DNA (genes) in a human cell

T. The joining of a part of or a whole chromosome to another separate chromosome

U. DNA sequences that are natural variations in a gene usually having no adverse effects on the individual

FOCUSED STUDY

1. Discuss the difference between mitosis and meiosis cell division. What role do they play in chromosomal alteration?

_____

_____

_____

_____

2. Explain the principles of inheritance and discuss how nurses can apply these principles when performing genetic counseling.

_____

_____

_____

_____

3. List specific examples of genetic testing and the condition, disease, or trait for which each test screens.

_____

_____

_____

_____

4. Discuss the importance of performing a thorough patient genetic intake and history. List items that must be included in a comprehensive genetic intake and history.

_____

_____

_____

_____

CASE STUDIES

Case Study 1

Janine Steinman, a 27-year-old married female, is being seen for her first prenatal visit by Dr. Williams. Mrs. Steinman reports that her relatives have a history of Tay-Sachs disease and that she is concerned about her child's potential for developing the disease. Dr. Williams orders a carrier test followed by genetic counseling. Answer the following questions based on your knowledge of Tay-Sachs disease and genetic implications.

1. Why did the physician order carrier testing for Mrs. Steinman?

2. How can the Steinmans be assured of the accuracy of their genetic testing results?

3. Who may obtain the results of the Steinmans' genetic testing?

CASE STUDY 2

Dianne Simmons, a 42-year-old female, is considering having an elective bilateral mastectomy. Ms. Simmons has a strong family history of breast cancer. Ms. Simmons's mother, sister, maternal aunt, and great-grandmother have all been diagnosed with and treated for breast cancer. Ms. Simmons is consulting with Dr. Powers and his team to determine whether an elective bilateral mastectomy will lessen the likelihood of her developing a form of breast cancer. Answer the following questions based on your knowledge of breast cancer and genetic implications.

1. Describe the predictive genetic testing that Ms. Simmons will have performed.

2. Why is it important to discuss and map Ms. Simmons's family tree in relation to breast cancer?

3. What type of nursing diagnoses will the nurse include in Ms. Simmons's genetic counseling care plan?

4. How can the testing information obtained by Ms. Simmons be used in the care of her extended family members?

CROSSWORD PUZZLE

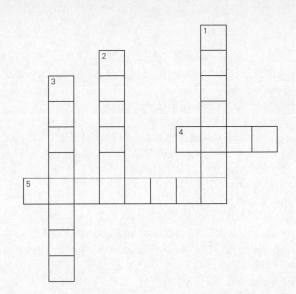

Across

4   The same

5   The loss of a single chromosome from a pair

Down

1   The gain of a single chromosome

2   Different

3   The normal number of 46 chromosomes

REVIEW QUESTIONS

1. A nurse is reviewing the patient's chromosomal report. What is the correct number of chromosomes per nucleus the nurse recognizes?

  1. 23

  2. 33

  3. 46

  4. 52

2. DNA molecules consist of long sequences of nucleotides or bases represented by what letters?

  1. A, G, T, and C

  2. A, H, P, and S

  3. T, O, D, and P

  4. A, D, S, and M

3. Down syndrome is better known as what?

  1. trisomy 5

  2. duosomy 19

  3. trisomy 21

  4. monosomic 16

4. The nurse is providing inheritance risk assessment and teaching to a patient. Which statement is incorrect?

  1. "A family history of multiple male miscarriages may be a sign of an X-linked recessive condition."

  2. "The sex chromosome X is unevenly distributed to males and females."

  3. "An individual with a recessive condition has inherited one altered gene from his or her mother and one from his or her father."

  4. "Homozygous-dominant conditions are generally more severe than heterozygous-dominant conditions and are often lethal."

5. A newborn undergoes what type of genetic newborn testing for phenylketonuria (PKU)?
   1. predictive genetic testing
   2. pharmacogenetic testing
   3. carrier testing
   4. newborn screening

6. The preceptor would correct which portion of a new nurse's plan of care for a patient who is to have genetic testing?
   1. Discuss risks and benefits of the testing.
   2. Assess for emotional stress caused by the testing and results.
   3. Investigate the cost of the procedure to be performed and its impact on family resources.
   4. Obtain verbal consent to avoid disclosing the patient's identity on a written consent.

7. A patient has a strong family history for the BRCA1 and BRCA2 tumor suppressor genes. What would be observed in the evaluation of successful genetic counseling in this patient?
   1. undergoes her first mammogram by age 50
   2. keeps the counseling session information private
   3. begins early clinical breast screenings at a young age
   4. does not perform breast self-exams due to unlikelihood of feeling these tumors

8. Mitochondrial genes and any diseases due to DNA alterations on those genes are transmitted by what means?
   1. through the mother in a matrilineal pattern
   2. through the father in a patrilineal pattern
   3. by either parent
   4. Mitochondrial diseases are not transmitted based on a sex link.

9. A genetic counselor has just informed a female patient that carrier testing has confirmed that she, her husband, and her infant daughter are positive for the sickle cell trait. The nurse would be most surprised if the patient expressed which emotion?
   1. survivor guilt
   2. fear
   3. shame
   4. self-image disturbance

Nursing Care of Patients in **Pain**

LEARNING OUTCOMES

1. Explain the neurophysiology of pain.
2. Compare and contrast definitions and characteristics of acute, chronic, central, and phantom pain.
3. Discuss factors affecting individualized responses to pain.
4. Describe interprofessional care for the patient in pain, including medications, surgery, transcutaneous electrical nerve stimulation, and complementary therapies.

CLINICAL COMPETENCIES

1. Use clinical reasoning to provide individualized nursing care for patients experiencing pain.
2. Assess patients' pain intensity, quality, location, pattern, intensifiers, relievers; side effects of analgesics; and effect on function and mood.
3. Determine patient's expressed desire, values, preference, and support for pain management.
4. In collaboration with the healthcare team, intervene with appropriate evidence-based nursing measures to promote patient comfort and include pharmacologic and nonpharmacologic methodologies.
5. Revise the plan of care according to the patient's response to interventions and need for control.
6. Use equianalgesia tables to select and transition between opioid analgesics.
7. Teach patients about safe and effective self-management of pain.
8. Evaluate the effectiveness of interventions to relieve pain and promote comfort; retreat or adjust doses of medication and interventions as necessary.

TERMS MATCHING

Place the letter of the correct definition in the space next to each term

1. _____ acute pain

2. _____ addiction

3. _____ analgesic

4. _____ breakthrough pain

5. _____ chronic pain

6. _____ equianalgesic

7. _____ neuropathic pain

8. _____ nociceptive pain

9. _____ nociceptors

10. _____ pain

11. _____ titrate

A. To increase or decrease medication doses in small increments

B. Prolonged pain, usually lasting longer than 6 months, or pain that persists after the condition causing it has resolved

C. Has sudden onset, is usually self-limited, and is localized; lasts for less than 6 months and has an identifiable cause, such as trauma, surgery, or inflammation

D. A medication that reduces or eliminates the perception of pain

E. Pain caused by stimulation of peripheral or visceral pain receptors

F. Approximate equivalent doses of opioid analgesics as compared to morphine sulfate

G. Sensory nerve fibers that conduct pain impulses from the periphery to the central nervous system

H. Discomfort that exceeds baseline levels of discomfort; often described as a sudden flare that exceeds the analgesic effect of long-acting pain medications

I. A primary, chronic neurobiologic disease characterized by compulsive use of a substance despite negative consequences such as health threats or legal problems

J. A subjective response to both physical and psychologic stressors

K. Caused by stimulation of peripheral or visceral pain receptors

FOCUSED STUDY

1. Describe the differences between acute and chronic pain.

_____

_____

_____

_____

2. List factors that influence a patient's response to pain.

_____

_____

_____

_____

3. Describe the different methods of administering medication.

_____

_____

_____

_____

4. What are the nurse's responsibilities when educating a patient who uses NSAIDs to help control pain?

_____

_____

_____

_____

CASE STUDIES

Case Study 1

John Browning was brought to the emergency room after suffering a traumatic amputation of his right lower leg during a motor vehicle accident. An emergency above-knee amputation was performed soon after his arrival at the hospital.

1. Which nerve fibers will transmit pain sensations from John Browning's injury to his spinal cord?

2. What form of acute pain will he experience immediately after the injury?

3. Which type of pain is Mr. Browning most at risk for developing as a result of his injuries?

4. What strategies will the nurse employ to best assess Mr. Browning's pain?

Case Study 2

Bailey Bowen is a 32-year-old male who suffers from recurrent lower back pain as a result of an injury that occurred at work. Mr. Bowen is a construction worker. Mr. Bowen has come to the physician's office for pain relief.

1. What factors will influence Mr. Bowen's perceived level of pain?

2. What strategies other than medication administration can be used to lessen Mr. Bowen's perceived level of pain?

3. What types of medications would you expect this patient to be prescribed for pain control at home?

4. Mr. Bowen's doctor has discussed placing a transcutaneous electrical nerve stimulation (TENS) unit on the patient. Explain how this may benefit a patient with chronic pain.

CROSSWORD PUZZLE

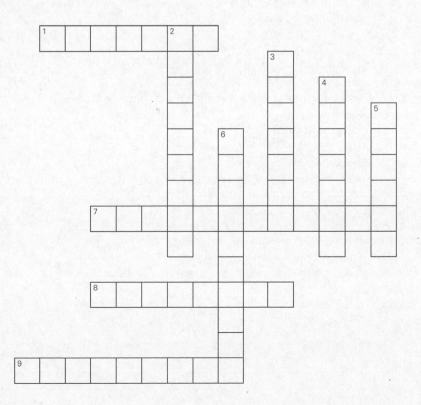

Across

1 The "Q" of the PQRST mnemonic
7 Dull, poorly localized pain arising from body organs
8 Another name for an opioid analgesic
9 The dorsal spinal roots are severed during this type of surgery

Down

2 The amount of pain a person can endure before outwardly responding to the pain
3 A brand name of an analgesic that should be avoided if the patient has a history of alcohol abuse
4 A type of pain with associated changes in sensations that is caused by a lesion or damage to the brain or spinal cord
5 The "T" of the PQRST mnemonic
6 A surgery used to remove or destroy a nerve

REVIEW QUESTIONS

1. The patient is complaining of nausea and a deep cramping pain in the abdomen. The patient is unable to localize the pain. The patient is most likely experiencing what type of pain?
   1. somatic pain
   2. visceral pain
   3. referred pain
   4. hyperesthesia pain

2. When caring for a geriatric patient, the nurse is aware of which fact?
   1. As a patient ages, the perception of pain decreases.
   2. Opioids cause excessive respiratory depression in older adults.
   3. Older adult patients fear narcotic addiction.
   4. Pain is a part of growing older.

3. Which statement is a common misconception regarding pain?
   1. Pain is a condition and not just a symptom.
   2. Narcotic medication is an appropriate method to help relieve a patient's chronic pain.
   3. Patients rarely lie about their pain.
   4. Pain relief interferes with a healthcare provider's ability to diagnose the source of the patient's pain.

4. The patient has been diagnosed with herpes zoster. The nurse is aware that pain control may be best achieved by administering a medication from which class?
   1. local anesthetics
   2. anticonvulsants
   3. narcotics
   4. nonsteroidal anti-inflammatory drugs (NSAIDs)

5. What is an advantage of administering pain medication before the patient experiences pain?
   1. The patient may spend less time in pain.
   2. Frequent administration allows for larger doses.
   3. The patient's fear and anxiety about the return of pain will increase.
   4. The patient will be less physically active.

6. The patient has been ordered a transdermal analgesic patch. Which statement demonstrates that the patient understands the use and application of the patch?
   1. "I will change this patch every 24 hours."
   2. "I should apply it in the same place each time I reapply a new patch."
   3. "A heating pad may increase how fast I absorb the medication."
   4. "I can expect to feel pain relief 10 hours after I apply the patch."

7. The patient is experiencing pain. Which finding would the nurse characterize as unexpected?
   1. shallow, rapid breathing
   2. increased blood pressure
   3. increased pulse rate
   4. constricted pupil

Nursing Care of Patients with **Altered Fluid, Electrolyte, and Acid–Base Balance**

LEARNING OUTCOMES

1. Describe the functions and regulatory mechanisms that maintain water, electrolyte, and acid–base balance in the body.
2. Compare and contrast the causes, pathophysiology, effects, and care of the patient with fluid volume or electrolyte imbalance.
3. Describe the causes, effects, and management of acid–base imbalances.

CLINICAL COMPETENCIES

1. Recognize patients at risk for fluid, electrolyte, or acid–base imbalances.
2. Assess and monitor fluid, electrolyte, and acid–base balance, communicating findings with appropriate interprofessional team members.
3. Demonstrate effective use of individualized and patient-centered strategies to reduce the risk of fluid, electrolyte, or acid–base imbalances.
4. Effectively communicate and function within the interprofessional team to plan and provide care to patients with altered fluid, electrolyte, and acid–base balance.
5. Administer fluids, medications, and other prescribed therapies knowledgeably and safely, using guideline or protocols as appropriate.
6. Adapt individual cultural values, expressed needs and preferences, and available evidence into the plan of care to provide knowledgeable and safe care to patients with fluid, electrolyte, or acid–base imbalances.
7. Use assessed data, patient values, and evidence to provide patient and family teaching about strategies to promote, restore, and maintain fluid, electrolyte, and acid–base balance.
8. Document care in the electronic medical record and use information management tools to monitor outcomes of care.
9. Participate in studies and projects to improve the quality and safety of care for patients with fluid, electrolyte, or acid–base disorders.

TERMS MATCHING

Place the letter of the correct definition in the space next to each term.

1. _____ acid

2. _____ acidosis

3. _____ alkalis

4. _____ alkalosis

5. _____ arterial blood gases (ABGs)

6. _____ atrial natriuretic peptide (ANP)

7. _____ base

8. _____ base excess (BE)

9. _____ dehydration

10. _____ edema

11. _____ fluid volume deficit (FVD)

12. _____ fluid volume excess

13. _____ homeostasis

14. _____ hypercapnia

15. _____ hypervolemia

16. _____ hypovolemia

17. _____ Kussmaul's respirations

18. _____ orthopnea

19. _____ serum bicarbonate

20. _____ tetany

21. _____ third spacing

A. The loss of water from the body

B. A decrease in interstitial, intravascular, and/or intracellular fluid in the body

C. A calculated value that reflects the degree of acid–base imbalance by indicating the status of the body's total buffering capacity

D. The body's tendency to maintain a state of physiologic balance in the presence of constantly changing conditions

E. The accumulation and sequestration of trapped extracellular fluid in an actual or potential body space as a result of disease or injury

F. Another term for bases; will accept hydrogen ions in solution

G. Excess accumulation of fluid in the interstitial spaces as a result of conditions that cause retention of sodium and water

H. HCO_3 reflects the renal regulation of acid–base balance; often called the metabolic component of arterial blood gases

I. Tonic muscular spasms that can be a result of hypocalcemia

J. Excess intravascular fluid

K. Deep and rapid respirations

L. Excess extracellular fluid resulting from retention of both water and sodium in the body

M. Condition in which the hydrogen ion concentration increases to an above-normal level (pH falls below 7.35)

N. Increased blood levels of carbon dioxide

O. A diagnostic test used to measure acid–base balance and gas exchange

P. Decreased circulating blood volume

Q. Condition in which the hydrogen ion concentration falls below normal (pH is above 7.45)

R. Difficulty breathing when lying down

S. Compound that releases hydrogen ions in solution

T. A hormone released by atrial muscle cells in response to distention from overload

U. Accepts hydrogen solutions in a solution

FOCUSED STUDY

1. Describe the differences between intracellular fluid (ICF) and extracellular fluid (ECF).

_____

_____

_____

_____

2. Describe the following ways that fluids move within the body:

a. Osmosis

_____

_____

b. Diffusion

_____

_____

c. Filtration

_____

_____

d. Active transport

_____

_____

3. Describe how each acid or base imbalance is produced.
   a. Metabolic acidosis and alkalosis

_____

_____

   b. Respiratory acidosis and alkalosis

_____

_____

4. List three expected outcomes for the patient who has been diagnosed with metabolic alkalosis.
   1. _____
   2. _____
   3. _____

CASE STUDY

Mr. Sweeney has been admitted with diabetic ketoacidosis. The patient's arterial blood gas values are abnormal. Answer the following questions based on his diagnosis.

1. Which acid–base imbalance is this patient most at risk for developing?

2. What is a normal pH? What does the nurse expect Mr. Sweeney's pH to be based on his admitting diagnosis and abnormal arterial blood gas values?

3. The nurse would expect Mr. Sweeney's respirations to be of what quality and depth? What is the specific name for this type of breathing?

4. What are the early manifestations of this type of acid–base imbalance?

5. As the nurse reviews the results of this patient's laboratory tests, what are the expected changes that may be seen in potassium and magnesium levels?

6. What are vital teaching areas for Mr. Sweeney?

7. How is the heart's ability to function affected by this type of acid–base imbalance?

SHORT ANSWERS

Fill in the following table.

Condition	Laboratory Values	Short Questions Regarding Clinical Manifestations	Answer
Hyponatremia		Has this patient's blood pressure increased or decreased?	
Hypernatremia		Has this patient gained or lost weight?	
Hypokalemia		Hypokalemia increases the patient's risk of developing toxicity related to which medication?	

Condition	Laboratory Values	Short Questions Regarding Clinical Manifestations	Answer
Hyperkalemia		Which medication may be ordered to increase renal potassium excretion?	
Hypocalcemia		When should the hypocalcemic patient be instructed to take his or her ordered oral calcium salts?	
Hypercalcemia		Will the hyperkalemic patient develop muscle weakness or tetany?	
Hypomagnesemia		This patient is receiving intravenous magnesium sulfate. The function of which organ should be monitored during this type of therapy?	
Hypermagnesemia		Will deep tendon reflexes be hyperactive or hypoactive in a patient with this condition?	
Hypophosphatemia		Nursing interventions for this patient should be focused on which types of issues?	
Hyperphosphatemia		Is this patient more likely to suffer from complications related to hypotension or hypertension?	

REVIEW QUESTIONS

1. What substance can be immediately replaced intravascularly?
   1. plasma
   2. urine
   3. synovial fluid
   4. perspiration
2. Identify the primary process that controls body fluid movement between the intracellular fluid (ICF) and extracellular fluid (ECF) compartments.
   1. osmosis
   2. diffusion
   3. active transport
   4. filtration
3. Monitoring what finding in the older adult is a poor indicator of fluid volume deficit?
   1. skin turgor
   2. tongue furrows
   3. blood pressure
   4. weight
4. A patient is diagnosed with fluid volume deficit due to a severe burn injury. What laboratory finding would be unexpected?
   1. decrease in potassium
   2. elevated hemoglobin
   3. increase in urine specific gravity
   4. decreased hematocrit
5. What is the initial clinical manifestation associated with hypernatremia?
   1. lethargy
   2. weakness
   3. thirst
   4. irritability
6. A buffer prevents major changes in pH by releasing what type of ions?
   1. hydrogen
   2. calcium
   3. sodium
   4. magnesium

Nursing Care of Patients Experiencing Trauma and Shock

LEARNING OUTCOMES

1. Define the word *trauma*.
2. Define the components and types of trauma.
3. Describe the result of energy transfer to the human body.
4. Discuss causes, effects, and initial management of trauma.
5. Discuss diagnostic tests used in assessing patients experiencing trauma and shock.
6. Describe collaborative interventions for patients experiencing trauma and shock, including medications, blood transfusion, and intravenous fluids.
7. Discuss organ donation and forensic implications of traumatic injury or death.
8. Discuss cellular homeostasis and basic hemodynamics.
9. Discuss the risk factors, etiologies, and pathophysiologies of hypovolemic shock, cardiogenic shock, obstructive shock, and distributive shock.
10. Use the nursing process as a framework for providing individualized care to patients experiencing trauma and shock.

CLINICAL COMPETENCIES

1. Describe steps of the primary survey to diagnose and manage life-threatening injuries.
2. Obtain initial subjective and objective data of the trauma patient to include history taking, assessment, review of past medical history, and communication with pre-hospital and other healthcare providers and family members.
3. Evaluate patient response to medical and surgical interventions for patients sustaining multiple trauma and shock.
4. Provide essential ongoing written communication for patient care and continuity of the trauma patient.
5. Describe the role of the nurse in trauma prevention education and develop a plan of care to restore the functional health status of trauma patients.
6. Communicate significant data and changes in the condition of a patient who has sustained trauma.
7. Identify nursing diagnoses based on signs and symptoms recognized during the nursing assessment.
8. Develop a plan of care for the trauma patient based on scientific knowledge and patient diversity that addresses the nursing diagnosis.
9. Document quality of care issues associated with the trauma patient.
10. Advocate for the patient's rights as indicated by documents that address end-of-life issues.
11. Comply with guidelines related to the Uniform Anatomical Gift Act.

TERMS MATCHING

Place the letter of the correct definition in the space next to each term.

1. _____ abrasion
2. _____ brain death criteria
3. _____ contusion
4. _____ laceration
5. _____ pneumothorax
6. _____ puncture wound
7. _____ shock
8. _____ tension pneumothorax
9. _____ transfusion
10. _____ trauma

A. A systemic imbalance between oxygen supply and demand that results in a state of inadequate blood flow to body organs and tissues, causing life-threatening cellular dysfunction

B. An open wound that is the result of a sharp cut or tear

C. Results when air enters the pleural space due to blunt and penetrating injuries to the chest

D. Clinical signs used to determine whether a comatose patient is brain dead

E. An infusion of blood or blood components

F. Injury to human tissue and organs that is the result of a transfer of energy from the environment

G. A partial-thickness denudation of an area of integument, usually occurring as the result of a fall or scrape

H. A condition in which an injury to the chest allows air to enter but not escape the pleural cavity

I. A superficial tissue injury that is the result of blunt trauma; small blood vessels break, and there is bleeding into the surrounding tissues

J. Wound that occurs when a sharp or blunt object penetrates the integument

FOCUSED STUDY

1. List factors that may influence the host's susceptibility to injury during a traumatic event.

_____

_____

_____

2. When caring for a patient with a possible cervical spine injury, what five criteria indicate that the patient probably did not experience a cervical spine injury?

   a.

   _____

   b.

   _____

   c.

   _____

   d.

   _____

   e.

   _____

3. Which blood type is known as the "universal recipient"? Which blood type is known as the "universal donor"?

   Universal recipient _____

   Universal donor _____

4. According to the Uniform Anatomical Gift Act, who may give consent for organ donation?

   _____

   _____

   _____

CASE STUDY

Mr. Richard Key, a 26-year-old male, was involved in a motorcycle accident along a rural road. A passing motorist found him lying next to a tree and his motorcycle. Mr. Key was unconscious. Answer the following questions based on your knowledge about the care of a patient who has suffered trauma.

1. What types of trauma did Mr. Key potentially experience?

2. What method of transportation will most likely be used to transport Mr. Key to the hospital? To what trauma level hospital should he be transported?

3. As healthcare providers assess Mr. Key, what is their highest priority?

4. What diagnostic studies may be performed on Mr. Key once he reaches the trauma center?

5. The physician notes that Mr. Key has developed a tension pneumothorax. What clinical manifestations are associated with this diagnosis?

6. After several days, healthcare providers determine that Mr. Key has experienced brain death. The family wants to donate his organs. Mr. Key is found to be an ineligible donor. What are some possible reasons for this?

7. What criteria are used to determine that Mr. Key has experienced brain death?

REVIEW QUESTIONS

1. What type of energy is most commonly transferred to a host in trauma?
   1. mechanical
   2. gravitational
   3. thermal
   4. electrical
2. The nurse receives a report that the incoming patient has suffered a minor trauma. Which injury would the nurse classify as a minor trauma?
   1. gunshot wound
   2. compression injury
   3. stab wound
   4. fractured clavicle
3. Identify the organ system that is not involved in multiple organ dysfunction syndrome (MODS).
   1. reproductive
   2. pulmonary
   3. hepatic
   4. cardiovascular
4. The patient has been admitted to the hospital with multiple trauma. Which medication order would the nurse question?
   1. opioids
   2. vasodilators
   3. inotropic drugs
   4. crystalloids
5. A patient is experiencing shock. What clinical manifestation would the nurse not expect to find during the assessment?
   1. apical heart rate of 122 beats per minute
   2. increased carbon dioxide levels
   3. hyperactive bowel sounds and diarrhea
   4. cerebral hypoxia
6. What type of shock is the leading cause of death for patients in intensive care units?
   1. hypovolemic shock
   2. septic shock
   3. cardiogenic shock
   4. neurogenic shock
7. The nurse is administering a blood transfusion. The nurse knows that the goal of blood administration is to keep the hematocrit in what range?
   1. from 20%–25%
   2. from 30%–35%
   3. from 40%–45%
   4. from 50%–55%

CHAPTER 12

Nursing Care of Patients with **Infection**

LEARNING OUTCOMES

1. Explain the components and functions of the immune system and the immune response.
2. Compare antibody-mediated and cell-mediated immune responses.
3. Describe the pathophysiology of wound healing, inflammation, and infection.
4. Identify factors responsible for and the implications of healthcare-associated infections.
5. Discuss the purposes, nursing implications, and health education for medications and treatments used to treat inflammations and infections.
6. Explain the nursing care necessary to prevent and/or monitor the status of infections.

CLINICAL COMPETENCIES

1. Apply standard precautions and evidence-based practices to prevent the spread of infection within the patient, to other patients in the facility, and to members of the interprofessional team and visitors.
2. Provide safe, effective, and respectful patient-centered care for patients with inflammation and infection.
3. Collaborate with the interprofessional care team to integrate care of patients with infections.
4. Promote therapeutic levels and complete dosage of anti-inflammatory and anti-infective medication through prompt administration and patient and family teaching.
5. Assess for hypersensitivities to anti-inflammatory and anti-infective medication prior to and during administration.
6. Participate in quality improvement processes to reduce the rates and risk of infection for a patient group or population.

TERMS MATCHING

Place the letter of the correct definition in the space next to each term.

1. _____ abscess
2. _____ acquired immunity
3. _____ active immunity
4. _____ adaptive immune response
5. _____ anergy
6. _____ antibodies
7. _____ antibody-mediated (humoral) immune response
8. _____ antigen
9. _____ B lymphocytes (B cells)
10. _____ cell-mediated (cellular) immune response
11. _____ cytokines
12. _____ endotoxins
13. _____ exotoxins
14. _____ healthcare-associated infections (HAIs)
15. _____ immunity
16. _____ immunocompetent
17. _____ immunoglobulin (Ig)
18. _____ infection
19. _____ inflammation
20. _____ innate immunity
21. _____ lymphocyte
22. _____ macrophages
23. _____ natural killer (NK) cells
24. _____ passive immunity
25. _____ pathogens
26. _____ phagocytosis
27. _____ septicemia
28. _____ T lymphocytes (T cells)
29. _____ vaccines

A. Infections acquired in a healthcare setting; also called nosocomial infections

B. Activation of B cells to produce antibodies to respond to antigens such as bacteria, bacterial toxins, and free viruses

C. A substance capable of evoking a specific immune response; usually a protein which the body recognizes as foreign, causing an immune response to be stimulated

D. Hormone-like polypeptides produced primarily by monocytes, macrophages, and T cells

E. A localized collection of pus

F. Found in the cell wall of gram-negative bacteria and released only when the cell is disrupted

G. One type of lymphocyte; part of the innate immune system, it provides immune surveillance and infection resistance, and plays an important role in the destruction of early malignant cells

H. Immunity developed after exposure to a pathogen

I. A nonspecific, generic response to tissue injury

J. Production of antibodies or development of immune lymphocytes against specific antigens.

K. A protein that functions as an antibody

L. Temporary protection against disease-producing antigens; the type of immunity that is provided by antibodies produced by other people or animals

M. The protection of the body from disease

N. A specific and systemic immune response initiated by and directed against particular antigens

O. Highly poisonous soluble proteins that are secreted into surrounding tissue by the microorganism

P. Direct or indirect inactivation of antigen by lymphocytes

Q. Inability to react to specific antigens

R. One type of lymphocyte that matures in the thymus gland

S. Immunoglobulin molecules that bind with an antigen and inactivate it

T. Colonization by and multiplication of an organism within a host

U. Bursa-equivalent lymphocytes responsible for synthesizing antibodies in response to specific antigens

V. Virulent organisms rarely found in the absence of disease

W. Possessing an immune system that can identify antigens and effectively destroy or remove them

X. A process by which a foreign agent or target cell is engulfed, destroyed, and digested; neutrophils and macrophages are the primary cells involved

Y. Suspensions of whole or fractionated bacteria or viruses that have been treated to make them nonpathogenic

Z. Mature monocytes that have settled into the tissues of the body

AA. A complex, nonspecific, adaptive response to injury that brings fluid, dissolved substances, and blood cells into the interstitial tissues where the invasion or damage has occurred

BB. The principal effector and regulator cells of specific immune responses

CC. Systemic disease associate with the presence of bacteria or their toxins in the blood

FOCUSED STUDY

1. Describe the location and function of the following lymphoid tissues.
   a. Spleen

   _____

   _____

   b. Thymus gland

   _____

   _____

   c. Bone marrow

   _____

   _____

2. Provide one example of acquired immunity and one example of passive immunity.
   a. Acquired immunity

   _____

   _____

   b. Passive immunity

   _____

   _____

3. Identify the usual indicators of inflammation. How are the clinical manifestations of an infection altered in the older adult?

   _____

   _____

   _____

   _____

4. Explain why the administration of antibiotics is ineffective in treating viral pathogens.

   _____

   _____

CASE STUDY

Sally Chase, a 12-year-old patient, is being seen in the clinic this morning. She is complaining of a sore throat and headache. Upon examination, her throat is found to be reddened with pustules present on each tonsil. After receiving diagnostic test results, the physician has prescribed penicillin. Sally has a streptococcal infection that is sensitive to penicillin. Answer the following questions based on your knowledge regarding the care of patients with infections.

1. What should the nurse include when educating Sally about taking penicillin?

2. What test was performed to identify the organism that is causing Sally's infection?

3. What are the important concerns the nurse should consider when creating Sally's care plan?

4. While taking penicillin, what types of things should Sally or her parents report to the physician?

5. Sally is presenting to the physician's office in which stage of the infectious process?

6. If this streptococcal throat infection is prolonged, what specific health problems may Sally be at an increased risk for developing?

SHORT ANSWERS

Fill in the table identifying the major chemical mediators of inflammation.

Factor	Source	Effect
Histamine		
Kinins (bradykinin and others)		
Prostaglandins		
Leukotrienes		

REVIEW QUESTIONS

1. Identify a function of the vascular response.
   1. Leukocytes marginate and emigrate into the damaged tissue.
   2. It is a process by which a foreign agent or target cell is engulfed, destroyed, and digested.
   3. It involves the introduction of antigens into the body.
   4. It localizes invading bacteria and keeps them from spreading.
2. Identify the correct statement about vaccines.
   1. Vaccines are suspensions of whole or fractionated bacteria or viruses that have been treated to make them pathogenic.
   2. Vaccines are administered to reduce an immune response.
   3. All vaccines are completely effective and entirely safe.
   4. Vaccines stimulate active immunity by inducing the production of antibodies and antitoxins.
3. Which statement demonstrates that the patient understands self-care activities that can be used to promote healing?
   1. "I must restrict my intake of water."
   2. "I have to stay as active as possible."
   3. "I will eat a well-balanced diet."
   4. "I should take an anti-inflammatory medication at the first sign of swelling."
4. The nurse is explaining to the student nurse the nursing interventions that can be used to help promote tissue integrity. Which nursing intervention would be questioned by the student nurse?
   1. Clean inflamed tissue gently.
   2. Keep the inflamed area moist and prevent exposure to air as much as possible.
   3. Balance rest with the tolerable degree of mobility.
   4. Provide protection and support for inflamed tissue.
5. Identify the most common type of healthcare-associated infection.
   1. urinary tract infection
   2. pneumonia
   3. bacteremia
   4. *Clostridium difficile*–associated diarrhea
6. The nurse is assessing the patient for an opportunistic infection. Which finding would be unexpected?
   1. complaints of constipation
   2. fuzzy growth on the tongue
   3. increased vaginal discharge
   4. blood in the urine

CHAPTER 13

Nursing Care of Patients with **Altered Immunity**

LEARNING OUTCOMES

1. Review the normal immune system function, including self-recognition.
2. Compare and contrast the four types of hypersensitivity reactions.
3. Explain the pathophysiology of autoimmune disorders and tissue transplant rejection.
4. Discuss the characteristics of immunodeficiencies.
5. Identify laboratory and diagnostic tests used to diagnose and monitor immune response.
6. Describe interprofessional therapies and medications used to treat patients with altered immunity.
7. Correlate the pathophysiological alterations with the manifestations of HIV/AIDS infection.

CLINICAL COMPETENCIES

1. Assess functional health status of patients with altered immunity and monitor, document, and report unexpected manifestations and responses.
2. Function competently within own scope of practice as a member of the healthcare team caring for patients with altered immune function.
3. Demonstrate sensitivity and respect for expressed values, culture, and preferences when planning and providing individualized and evidence-based care for individuals with altered immune responses.
4. Apply quality measures and best practices in caring for patients with altered immune responses.
5. Demonstrate effective strategies to reduce the risk of harm when caring for patients with altered immune responses.
6. Apply technology and information management tools to support safe care for patients with altered immune responses.

TERMS MATCHING

Place the letter of the correct definition in the space next to each item.

1. _____ acquired immunodeficiency syndrome (AIDS)

2. _____ allergy

3. _____ allograft

4. _____ anaphylaxis

5. _____ antigenic substances

6. _____ autograft

7. _____ autoimmune disorder

8. _____ histocompatibility

9. _____ human immunodeficiency virus (HIV)

10. _____ hypersensitivity

11. _____ immunosuppression

12. _____ Kaposi's sarcoma (KS)

13. _____ seroconversion

A. Agents such as microorganisms, cells and tissues from other humans or animals, and some inorganic substances that stimulate an immune response

B. A retrovirus first isolated in 1984, it is transmitted by direct contact with infected blood and body fluids; responsible for AIDS

C. Inability of the immune system to respond to an antigen. Occurs in response to disease or medications; may be intentional to prevent rejection of transplants or a side effect of some medications

D. Failure of immune system to recognize itself, resulting in normal host tissue being targeted by immune defenses

E. Exaggerated response of the immune system; allergies are an example of this type of problem

F. A tumor of the endothelial cells lining small blood vessels; presents as vascular macules, papules, or brown or violet lesions affecting the skin and viscera; associated with HIV infection

G. A transplant of the patient's own tissue

H. Antibody response to a disease or vaccine

I. A hypersensitive or altered immune response to an environmental or exogenous antigen

J. The ability of cells and tissues to survive transplantation without immunologic interference by the recipient; determined by tissue typing

K. Organ and tissue transplants between members of the same species but who have different genotypes and human leukocyte antigens

L. Acute systemic type I hypersensitivity reaction that occurs in response to an injected antigen

M. A specific group of diseases or conditions that are indicative of severe immunosuppression related to infection with the human immuno-deficiency virus

FOCUSED STUDY

1. Describe the differences among the following types of transplanted tissue rejection.
   a. Hyperacute tissue rejection:

   _____

   _____

   b. Acute tissue rejection:

   _____

   _____

   c. Chronic tissue rejection: _____

   _____

   _____

   d. Graft-versus-host disease:

   _____

   _____

2. Provide one example for each type of hypersensitivity response. Note whether each type is due to an antigen–antibody or antigen–lymphocyte interaction.
   a. Type I IgE-mediated hypersensitivity

   Example: _____

   Type of interaction: _____

b. Type II cytotoxic hypersensitivity

Example: _____

Type of interaction: _____

c. Type III immune complex

Example: _____

Type of interaction: _____

d. Type IV delayed hypersensitivity

Example: _____

Type of interaction: _____

3. When caring for a patient who has developed an anaphylactic reaction and has ineffective airway clearance, describe interventions that should be implemented.

_____

_____

_____

_____

4. List medications that can be used to treat the clinical manifestations associated with hypersensitivity reactions. Briefly list the intended action of each medication.

_____

_____

_____

CASE STUDIES

Case Study 1

Gary Jones is a 25-year-old African American homosexual who was recently diagnosed with AIDS. Answer the following questions based on your knowledge of caring for patients with HIV and AIDS.

1. What are Mr. Jones's specific risk factors for acquiring HIV?

2. How long after exposure would the nurse expect seroconversion to occur in Mr. Jones?

3. A few weeks ago Mr. Jones had nausea, diarrhea, and abdominal cramping. What might this indicate to the nurse?

4. Which opportunistic infections are associated with AIDS?

Case Study 2

Susan Callahan is a registered nurse who has developed contact dermatitis. The hospital where Susan works stocks powdered latex gloves. Susan has been newly diagnosed with a latex allergy. Answer the following questions based on your knowledge of caring for a patient with a latex allergy.

1. Besides latex gloves, what other items commonly made of latex may have contributed to Susan's allergy to latex?

2. How can employers protect their employees from developing latex allergies?

3. Susan wants to know why powdered latex gloves are "worse" than powder-free latex gloves for people with a latex sensitivity. How should the nurse caring for Susan answer this question?

4. If Susan developed a type I systemic allergic reaction as a result of a respiratory exposure, which two diagnostic tests would Susan's nurse expect to see ordered?

SHORT ANSWERS

The nurse is assessing the patient's immune system. Describe the findings that may accompany a patient with an infection or an immune disorder.

General appearance	
Mucous membranes in nose and mouth	
Skin	
Lymph nodes (cervical, axillae, and groin)	
Joints	

REVIEW QUESTIONS

1. The patient is being screened for a hypersensitivity reaction. The nurse would question which order because it will provide the least amount of information about a hypersensitivity reaction?
    1. red blood cell (RBC) count
    2. blood type and crossmatch
    3. Coombs' direct
    4. complement assay
2. Which statement indicates that the patient understands the best way to manage hypersensitivity to bee venom?
    1. "If I take an antihistamine daily, it will prevent a reaction if I am stung."
    2. "If I use penicillin immediately after I am stung, it will stop a reaction."
    3. "I should carry a bee sting kit at all times so that I can have quick access to epinephrine."
    4. "If I take prednisone each day, it will prevent a hypersensitivity reaction."
3. Transplanted cadaver tissue is known as what type of graft?
    1. autograft
    2. isograft
    3. allograft
    4. xenograft
4. Identify the malignancy that is least likely to be associated with HIV/AIDS.
    1. non-Hodgkin's lymphoma
    2. Kaposi's sarcoma
    3. lung cancer
    4. invasive cervical cancer
5. The patient with HIV has developed a reddened blister due to frequent episodes of diarrhea. Identify the appropriate nursing intervention.
    1. Rub the skin directly over the blister to enhance circulation.
    2. Open and drain the blister.
    3. Apply heat to the area three times daily until healed.
    4. Encourage ambulation to increase circulation and maintain muscle tone.

CHAPTER 14

Nursing Care of Patients with **Cancer**

LEARNING OUTCOMES

1. Explain known carcinogens and carcinogenesis, and identify risk factors for cancer.
2. Compare the mechanisms and characteristics of normal cells with malignant cells.
3. Describe the physical and psychologic effects of cancer.
4. Describe and compare laboratory and diagnostic tests for cancer.
5. Discuss the role of chemotherapy in cancer treatment and classify chemotherapeutic agents.
6. Compare and contrast the role of surgery, radiation therapy, and biotherapy in the treatment of cancer.
7. Explain causes and discuss the nursing interventions for common oncologic emergencies.
8. Design an appropriate care plan for patients with cancer and their families regarding cancer diagnosis, treatment, and coping strategies.

CLINICAL COMPETENCIES

1. Perform focused and comprehensive assessments of the patient with cancer, including functional status, physical and psychologic needs, and expressed values and preferences.
2. Use assessed data to determine priority nursing diagnoses, select individualized nursing interventions, evaluate patient responses, and revise the plan of care as needed to promote, maintain, or restore functional health, and to alleviate suffering.
3. Provide effective care for patients with cancer, integrating planned nursing care with the interprofessional plan of care.
4. Use current evidence and patient preferences to plan and implement optimal nursing care for patients with cancer.
5. Plan and provide appropriate teaching for self-care of cancer-related and treatment-related symptoms, such as pain, nausea and vomiting, mucositis, fatigue, or anemia.
6. Use quality measures, processes, and tools to improve outcomes for patients with cancer.
7. Include cultural variation and diverse values in designing and implementing individualized plans of care for patients with cancer.
8. Demonstrate effective use of technology, current evidence, and care standards to reduce the risk of harm for patients with cancer.
9. Use technology to obtain high-quality healthcare information and plan, document, communicate, and coordinate care for patients with cancer.

TERMS MATCHING

Place the letter of the correct definition in the space next to each term.

1. _____ anaplasia
2. _____ biotherapy
3. _____ brachytherapy
4. _____ cachexia
5. _____ cancer
6. _____ carcinogenesis
7. _____ carcinogens
8. _____ cell cycle
9. _____ chemotherapy
10. _____ differentiation
11. _____ dysplasia
12. _____ hospice
13. _____ hyperplasia
14. _____ metaplasia
15. _____ metastasis
16. _____ neoplasm
17. _____ oncogene
18. _____ oncologic emergencies
19. _____ oncology
20. _____ proto-oncogenes
21. _____ radiation therapy
22. _____ tumor marker
23. _____ xerostomia

A. A group of complex diseases characterized by uncontrolled growth of abnormal cells

B. The use of cytotoxic medications to cure some types of cancers, to decrease tumor size and to prevent or treat suspected metastases

C. The regression of a cell to an immature or undifferentiated cell type

D. Malignant cells from the primary tumor travel through the blood or lymph to invade other tissues and organs of the body and form a secondary tumor

E. Enhancing a patient's immune response to modify the biologic processes that result in malignant cells

F. A protein molecule detectable in serum or other body fluids used as a biochemical indicator of the presence of a malignancy

G. An increase in the number or density of normal cells

H. The wasted appearance associated with people who have cancer

I. A change in the normal pattern of differentiation; dividing cells differentiate into cell types not normally found in that location in the body

J. Gene capable of triggering cancerous characteristics

K. A special component of home care, designed to provide medical, nursing, social, psychologic, and spiritual care for terminally ill patients and their families

L. Certain agents that cause mutations in cellular DNA and transform cells into cancer cells

M. The study of cancer

N. Emergency situations that arise when caring for patients diagnosed with cancer

O. The process by which normal cells are transformed into cancer cells

P. The loss of DNA control over differentiation occurring in response to adverse conditions; affected cells show abnormal variation in size, shape, and appearance and a disturbance in their usual arrangement

Q. A collection of cells that grows independently of the surrounding structures and has no physiological purpose

R. The four phases that occur during growth and development of a cell

S. The type of cancer treatment that consists of delivering ionizing radiation consisting of gamma rays and x-rays

T. A normal process occurring over many cell cycles that allows cells to specialize in certain tasks

U. Excessive dryness of the mucous membranes

V. A type of radiation therapy in which the source of radiation is placed directly into or adjacent to the tumor, a technique that delivers a high dose to the tumor and a lower dose to normal tissue

W. Normal genes that promote cell growth and repair

FOCUSED STUDY

1. How can a person modify his or her diet to help prevent the occurrence of cancer?

_____

_____

_____

_____

2. How does stress play a role in cancer development?

_____

_____

_____

3. Describe the differences between benign and malignant neoplasms (appearance, growth, and effect on surrounding tissue).

_____

_____

_____

4. Briefly describe the following methods used to treat cancer.
   a. Surgery as a primary treatment for cancer:

_____

_____

   b. Chemotherapy:

_____

_____

   c. Radiation:

_____

_____

   d. Biotherapy:

_____

_____

   e. Photodynamic therapy:

_____

_____

CASE STUDY

Donna Lee is a 54-year-old female who had a liposarcoma and associated lymph nodes removed. The tumor was graded as T4, N2b, M2. Answer the following questions based on your knowledge of caring for a patient with cancer.

1. Is Mrs. Lee's tumor malignant or benign?

2. From what tissue did this tumor arise?

3. What is the significance of a T4 grade?

4. What is the significance of a N2b grade?

5. What is the significance of a M2 grade?

6. What is the term used to describe a benign tumor originating from similar tissue?

SHORT ANSWERS

Indicate the type(s) of cancer associated with each virus.

Virus	Cancer
Herpes simplex virus types I and II (HSV-1 and HSV-2)	a. b. c.
Human cytomegalovirus (HCMV)	a. b.
Epstein-Barr virus (EBV)	a.
Human herpesvirus 6 (HHV-6)	a.
Hepatitis B virus (HBV)	a.
Papillomavirus	a. b.
Human T-cell lymphotropic viruses (HTLVs)	a. b. c.

REVIEW QUESTIONS

1. Which type of cancer should the nurse screen for more closely in men than in women patients?
   1. skin
   2. bladder
   3. lung
   4. thyroid

2. The patient has been newly diagnosed with cancer and is undergoing the first chemotherapy treatment. Which statement indicates that the patient understands an effect of chemotherapy?
   1. "I will not lose my hair."
   2. "My body will respond quicker to an infection."
   3. "I may lose my sense of taste."
   4. "I will become pregnant easily while undergoing chemotherapy."

3. The patient has been diagnosed with an anxiety disorder. Which finding by the nurse would be unexpected?
   1. direct eye contact
   2. hyperactivity
   3. trembling
   4. withdrawal

4. The patient has recently undergone a right radical mastectomy. Which behavior indicates that the patient has maintained a positive body image after surgery?
   1. The patient denies a change in physical body appearance.
   2. The patient is willing to look at the wound.
   3. The patient requests that no visitors be allowed in her room.
   4. The patient prefers that only nursing staff perform care to the affected area.

5. Mr. Packer has recently been diagnosed with cancer. Which oral hygiene practice should be avoided?
   1. using a soft-tipped toothbrush
   2. using an alcohol-based mouthwash
   3. soaking dentures in hydrogen peroxide
   4. using waxed dental floss

6. The patient may have developed tumor lysis syndrome. Which sign would the nurse expect to find?
   1. hypouricemia
   2. hyperphosphatemia
   3. hypokalemia
   4. hyponatremia

CHAPTER 15

Assessing the Integumentary System

LEARNING OUTCOMES

1. Describe the anatomy, physiology, and functions of the skin, hair, and nails.
2. Discuss factors that influence skin color.
3. Identify specific topics for a health history interview of the patient with problems involving the skin, hair, or nails.
4. Explain techniques for assessing the skin, hair, and nails.
5. Give examples of genetic disorders of the integumentary system.
6. Describe normal variations in assessment findings for the older adult.
7. Identify abnormal findings that may indicate impairment of the integumentary system.

CLINICAL COMPETENCIES

1. Complete a health history of the integumentary system incorporating an appraisal of psychosocial and physiologic issues.
2. Conduct and document a health history for patients who have or are at risk for alterations in the skin, hair, or nails.
3. Conduct and document a physical assessment of the integumentary system, demonstrating sensitivity and respect for the diversity of the human experience.
4. Monitor the results of diagnostic tests and communicate abnormal findings within the interprofessional team.

TERMS MATCHING

Place the letter of the correct definition in the space next to each term.

1. _____ alopecia
2. _____ cyanosis
3. _____ ecchymosis
4. _____ edema
5. _____ erythema
6. _____ hirsutism
7. _____ jaundice
8. _____ keratin
9. _____ melanin
10. _____ pallor
11. _____ sebum
12. _____ urticaria
13. _____ vitiligo

A. Often referred to as hives and manifests as patches of pale, itchy wheals in an erythematous area

B. Raised bluish or yellowish vascular lesions also referred to as bruises

C. A yellow-to-orange color visible in the skin and mucous membranes; it is most often the result of a hepatic disorder

D. Patches of white spots on the skin that result from a loss of melanocytes

E. Hair loss

F. Skin pigment that forms a protective shield to protect eratinocytes and nerve endings in the dermis from the damaging effects of ultraviolet light

G. A fibrous, water-repellent protein that gives the epidermis its tough protective quality

H. A bluish discoloration of the skin and mucous membranes due to oxygen deficiency

I. Paleness of the skin

J. Accumulation of fluid in the body's tissues

K. An oily substance secreted from glands that provides lubrication to the hair and skin

L. Increased growth of coarse hair, usually on the face and trunk

M. A reddening of the skin

FOCUSED STUDY

1. What factors are responsible for the pigmented color of an individual's skin?

_____

_____

_____

2. Identify the two primary skin layers and their functions.

_____

_____

_____

3. Illnesses may result in color changes in the skin. List two conditions associated with color changes.

_____

_____

_____

CASE STUDY

Forty-two-year-old Cassandra Messersmith was admitted to a medical surgical unit with a diagnosis of symptomatic bradycardia and hypotension. Her vital signs are as follows: heart rate 52, blood pressure 89/56, and respiratory rate 24. She denies pain at this time. Her past medical history is significant for a small basal cell carcinoma on the side of her nose. The lesion was surgically excised without complication 1 year ago.

During the morning assessment, the nurse observes a red scaly area with papules on the back of the patient's scalp at the base of the hairline. When the nurse questions the patient about the area, the patient states that it appeared about a week ago and that it bleeds occasionally when she brushes her hair. The nurse measures the area (which is 3 mm), completes the assessment, and makes certain the patient is comfortable. The nurse then documents the findings and calls the physician with the morning lab results.

1. Is the area on the back of the patient's scalp a recurrence of her basal cell carcinoma? Why or why not?

2. What risk factors increase the patient's risk of developing this type of skin disorder?

3. The lesion is located on the back of the patient's head, and she noticed it a week ago. The lesion is 3 mm in size now. Explain two types of biopsy that may be done on this lesion.

4. Is there a connection between the reason for the patient's admission and the lesion found on the back of her head?

SHORT ANSWERS

1. Fill in the labels for the blanks in the figure. Then compare your answers with Figure 15-1 on page 378 of your textbook.

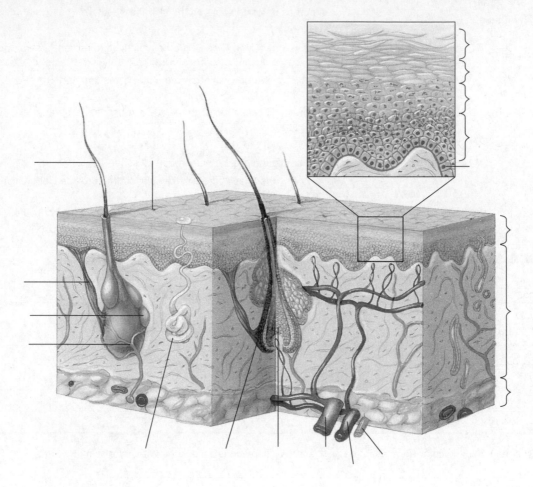

2. Fill in the labels for the blanks in the figure. Then compare your answers with Figure 15-3 on page 381 of your textbook.

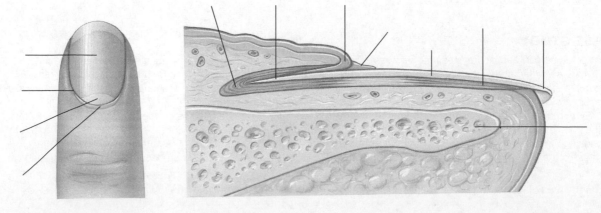

CROSSWORD PUZZLE

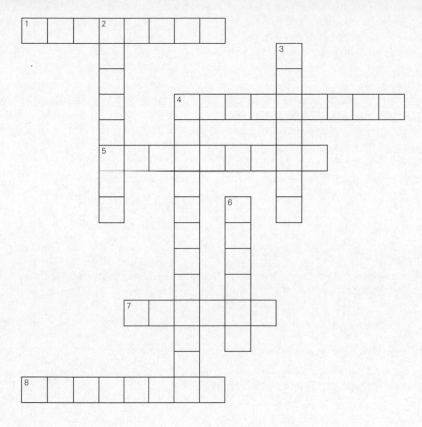

Across

1   Remnant of the sexual scent gland
4   Glands responsible for producing oil
5   The outermost surface of the skin
7   The second layer of skin
8   The total absence of melanin

Down

2   A yellow-to-orange pigment found in the body
3   Glands that regulate heat through perspiration
4   Glands responsible for the production of sweat
6   Retained urochrome pigments in the blood

REVIEW QUESTIONS

1. During a blood pressure screening, the nurse notices that the patient is scratching her abdomen. When the nurse asks about the scratching, the patient states that she has a red itchy rash under her breast. What is the most appropriate response from the nurse?
   1. "That happens in hot weather. It is probably just dry skin from bathing too much."
   2. "Scratching will only make it worse."
   3. "I think it is your new detergent. You should go back to what you were using before."
   4. "How long ago did the itching start?"

2. While assessing a patient, the nurse notices that the patient's ankles and feet are swollen to the point that her shoes are too tight. However, the skin slowly returns to normal when depressed by the nurse's thumb. This finding is most accurately documented as what?
   1. 1+
   2. 2+
   3. 3+
   4. 4+

3. A patient has a significantly receding hairline and a dark suntan. The nurse notices that he has a bandage on top of his head. When asked about it, he states that it is an odd mole that bleeds sometimes. Which of the following factors would increase the patient's risk of skin cancer?
    1. Smoked one pack of cigarettes a day for 15 years
    2. Worked as a landscaper for 10 years
    3. Consumed a high-fat diet
    4. Developed hypothyroidism

4. A nurse has been asked to speak to a community group about the risk factors associated with skin cancers. Which statement by the nurse would be most accurate?
    1. "A tendency to sunburn, even with sunscreen, increases your risk."
    2. "Family history is the strongest indicator of your risk."
    3. "Women have twice the risk of skin cancer as do men."
    4. "Your risk of skin cancer is less if you have a mild tan to the skin from a tanning bed."

5. When assessing a patient with dark skin color for jaundice, where is the best place to look?
    1. nail beds
    2. eyes
    3. forearm
    4. mucous membranes

6. The nurse notices that a patient is scratching her head. The nurse assesses the area and finds pustules and some hair loss. The nurse knows that these symptoms are associated with what?
    1. ringworm
    2. head lice
    3. seborrhea
    4. a boil

7. When assessing a patient's nails, the nurse notices that they are thick and yellow in color. The nurse knows that this is associated with which conditions? **Select all that apply.**
    1. fungal infection
    2. trauma to the nail
    3. pseudomonas infection
    4. psoriasis
    5. nutritional deficiency

8. When assessing the skin of a patient, the nurse notices that it is coarse. The nurse knows that coarse, dry skin is associated with what?
    1. hypothyroidism
    2. acne vulgaris
    3. fever
    4. seborrhea

Nursing Care of Patients with Integumentary Disorders

LEARNING OUTCOMES

1. Describe the manifestations, self-care, and nursing care of common skin problems and lesions.
2. Compare and contrast the etiology, pathophysiology, interprofessional care, and nursing care of patients with infections and infestations, inflammatory disorders, and malignancies of the skin.
3. Explain the risk factors for, pathophysiology of, and nursing interventions to prevent and care for pressure ulcers.
4. Discuss surgical options for excision of neoplasms, reconstruction of facial or body structures, and cosmetic procedures.
5. Explain the pathophysiology of selected disorders of the hair and nails.
6. Discuss the nursing implication related to the actions and effects of medications and other treatments for the patient with a disorder of the integumentary system.

CLINICAL COMPETENCIES

1. Assess the functional health status of patients with integumentary disorders and monitor, document, and report abnormal manifestations.
2. Plan and implement evidence-based nursing interventions for patients with pressure ulcers.
3. Consider assessment findings, patient values and beliefs, cultural norms, best practices, and clinical expertise when developing and implementing an individualized plan of care.
4. Apply safe practices during the administration of topical, oral, and injectable medications for the treatment of integumentary disorders.
5. Collaborate with the interprofessional team in the planning and provision of care for patients with integumentary disorders.
6. Implement patient teaching focused on prevention and management of integumentary disorders.
7. Revise the plan of care as needed to provide effective interventions to promote, maintain, or restore functional health status to patients with disorders of the integument.

TERMS MATCHING

Place the letter of the correct definition in the space next to each term.

1. _____ acne
2. _____ actinic keratosis
3. _____ angioma
4. _____ basal cell cancer
5. _____ carbuncle
6. _____ cellulitis
7. _____ comedones
8. _____ cysts
9. _____ dermatitis
10. _____ dermatophytoses
11. _____ folliculitis
12. _____ frostbite
13. _____ furuncle
14. _____ herpes simplex
15. _____ herpes zoster
16. _____ keloids
17. _____ keratosis
18. _____ lichen planus
19. _____ malignant melanoma
20. _____ nevi
21. _____ paronychia
22. _____ pemphigus vulgaris
23. _____ pressure ulcer
24. _____ pruritus
25. _____ psoriasis
26. _____ scabies
27. _____ skin graft
28. _____ squamous cell cancer
29. _____ warts
30. _____ xerosis

A. A bacterial infection of the hair follicle; most commonly caused by *Staphylococcus aureus*

B. A group of infected hair follicles

C. A localized infection of dermis and subcutaneous tissue

D. A subjective itching sensation producing an urge to scratch

E. Any skin condition in which there is a benign overgrowth and thickening of the cornified epithelium

F. A disorder of the pilosebaceous (hair and sebaceous gland) structure, resulting in eruption of papules or pustules

G. An injury of the skin as a result of freezing

H. Dry skin

I. A chronic disorder of the skin and oral mucous membranes caused by autoantibodies, resulting in blister formation

J. Superficial fungal skin infection; also called ringworm

K. Flat or raised macules or papules with rounded, well-defined borders; also known as moles

L. Benign closed sacs in or under the skin surface that are lined with epithelium and contain fluid or a semisolid material

M. A chronic immune skin disorder characterized by raised, reddened, round circumscribed plaques covered by silvery white scales

N. A parasitic infestation caused by a mite (*Sarcoptes scabiei*)

O. Also known as shingles, a viral infection of a dermatome section of the skin caused by varicella zoster

P. An epidermal skin lesion directly related to chronic sun exposure and photodamage

Q. An infection of the cuticle of the fingernails or toenails that often follows a minor trauma and secondary infection with staphylococci, streptococci, or *Candida*

R. Lesions of the skin caused by the human papillomavirus (HPV)

S. An epithelial tumor believed to originate either from the basal layer of the epidermis or from cells in the surrounding dermal structures

T. An inflammatory disorder of the mucous membranes and skin having no known cause but associated with exposure to drugs or to film processing chemicals

U. Benign vascular tumors

V. Noninflammatory acne lesions commonly called pimples, whiteheads, and blackheads

W. A surgical method of detaching skin from a donor site and placing it in a recipient site, where it develops a new blood supply from the base of the wound

X. A malignant tumor of the squamous epithelium of the skin or mucous membranes occurring most often on areas of skin exposed to ultraviolet rays and weather

Y. An acute or chronic inflammation of the skin characterized by erythema and pain or pruritus

Z. An inflammation of the hair follicle that often begins as folliculitis, but the infection spreads down the hair shaft, through the wall of the follicle, and into the dermis; may also be referred to as a boil

AA. A viral infection of the skin and mucous membranes (also called a fever blister or cold sore)

BB. Elevated, irregularly shaped, progressively enlarging scar that forms as a result of deposits of excessive amounts of collagen during scar formation

CC. A serious skin cancer that arises from melanocytes

DD. Ischemic lesions of the skin and underlying tissues caused by unrelieved pressure that impairs the flow of blood and lymph, resulting in tissue necrosis and eventual ulceration

FOCUSED STUDY

1. The nurse is instructing a patient about the rationale for prescribed therapeutic baths. What purpose do they serve for patients experiencing integumentary disorders?

_____

_____

_____

2. The nurse is preparing a therapeutic bath for a patient. When preparing the bath, what safety precautions should the nurse institute?

_____

_____

_____

_____

3. The nurse is evaluating a patient and documents the fact that the patient has a stage II pressure ulcer. What assessment findings will confirm this stage of pressure ulcer?

_____

_____

_____

4. The physician has prescribed Retin-A® to manage a patient's acne outbreaks. When providing education to the patient concerning this medication, what information should the nurse include?

_____

_____

_____

_____

CASE STUDY

Chrissy Green is a 30-year-old attorney with blonde hair and green eyes. She is very tan and reports a lot of sun exposure since childhood and notes that she frequently goes to a tanning booth "or I get so pale." She has been seen in the physician's office for a large, dark pigmented area on her right shoulder. The lesion is irregular in shape and has grown in size over the past year. Answer the following questions based on your knowledge of malignant melanoma.

1. What factors place Chrissy at risk for developing malignant melanoma?

2. What is Chrissy's prognosis? What factors are used to determine the prognosis?

3. What treatments are available to Chrissy?

4. How often must Chrissy be seen for a checkup after removal of the lesion?

SHORT ANSWERS

Review the following types of treatments used to manage integumentary disorders. Complete the table by listing indications and names of products used.

Type	Use	Examples
Creams		
Ointments		
Lotions		
Anesthetics		
Antibiotics		
Corticosteroids		

REVIEW QUESTIONS

1. Upon assessment, the nurse finds a skin lesion that looks like a flat or raised macule or papule with a rounded, well-defined border. The nurse suspects what type of diagnosis?
   1. cyst
   2. nevi
   3. keloid
   4. skin tag

2. The nurse is providing instructions for a patient who has psoriasis. When the nurse is discussing the patient's condition, which topics should be included? **Select all that apply**.
   1. Avoid exposure to the sun.
   2. Avoid exposure to contagious illnesses.
   3. Avoid trauma to the skin.
   4. Indomethacin and beta-adrenergic blocking agents are known to precipitate exacerbations of psoriasis.
   5. Avoid warm baths and showers.

3. Which behavior demonstrates the patient's understanding of the nurse's teaching about a vaginal *Candida albicans* infection?
   1. The patient inserts the prescribed intravaginal medication just inside the vagina.
   2. The patient wears silk or silk-lined underwear.
   3. The patient reports bathing more frequently.
   4. The patient reports not discussing the infection with her sexual partner.

4. Which form of dermatitis is a chronic inflammatory disorder of the skin that involves the scalp, eyebrows, eyelids, ear canals, nasolabial folds, axillae, and trunk?
   1. contact dermatitis
   2. atopic dermatitis
   3. seborrheic dermatitis
   4. exfoliative dermatitis

5. At what temperature does skin freeze?
   1. 0°F–10°F
   2. 14°F–24.8°F
   3. 32°F–50°F
   4. 55°F–72°F

6. The patient's medical record reports presence of a "venous lake" on the back of the right hand. The nurse would assess for which finding?
   1. small, bright red papule with radiating lines
   2. small, flat, blue lesion
   3. small, rounded red papule
   4. dark purple macular patch covering the hand

7. Identify the correct statement about skin grafts.
   1. A split-thickness graft contains only epidermis.
   2. A common donor site for a skin graft is the posterior thigh.
   3. Skin grafting is an effective way to cover wounds that are infected.
   4. A full-thickness graft is best able to withstand trauma.

Nursing Care of Patients with Burns

LEARNING OUTCOMES

1. Discuss the types and causative agents of burns.
2. Explain burn classification by depth and extent of injury.
3. Compare and contrast the pathophysiology and interprofessional care of a minor burn and a major burn.
4. Discuss the systemic pathophysiologic effects of a major burn and the stages of burn wound healing.
5. Explain the interprofessional care and nursing implications necessary during the emergent/resuscitative stage, the acute stage, and the rehabilitative stage of a major burn.

CLINICAL COMPETENCIES

1. Assess the functional health status of patients with burns, and monitor, document, and report abnormal manifestations.
2. Use evidence-based practice to plan and implement nursing care for patients with burns.
3. Determine priority nursing diagnoses, based on assessed data, to select and implement individualized nursing interventions for patient with burns.
4. Administer medications knowledgeably and safely to patients with burns.
5. Integrate interprofessional care into the care of patients with burns.
6. Provide teaching appropriate for prevention of burns.
7. Revise the plan of care as needed to provide effective interventions to promote, maintain, or restore functional health status to patients with burns.

TERMS MATCHING

Place the letter of the correct definition in the space next to each term.

1. _____ allograft

2. _____ autografting

3. _____ burn.

4. _____ burn shock

5. _____ compartment syndrome

6. _____ contractures

7. _____ Curling's ulcers

8. _____ debridement

9. _____ eschar

10. _____ escharotomy

11. _____ fascial excision

12. _____ fasciectomy

13. _____ fluid resuscitation

14. _____ full-thickness burn

15. _____ heterograft

16. _____ homograft

17. _____ hypertrophic scar

18. _____ keloid

19. _____ partial-thickness burn

20. _____ superficial burn

21. _____ surgical debridement

22. _____ xenograft

A. A hard crust that forms during the acute stage of an injury. This crust covers the wound and harbors necrotic tissue

B. Grafts between members of the same species but who have different genotypes and HLA antigens

C. Replacement of the extensive fluid and electrolyte losses associated with major burn injuries

D. A burn that involves all layers of the skin, including the epidermis, dermis, and epidermal appendages; may extend into the subcutaneous fat, connective tissue, muscle, and bone

E. Acute ulcerations of the stomach or duodenum that form following a burn injury

F. An overgrowth of dermal tissue that remains within the boundaries of a wound

G. Elevated, irregularly shaped, progressively enlarging scar arising from excessive amounts of collagen in the stratum corneum during scar formation in connective tissue repair

H. Transplanting of the patient's own tissue; the most successful type of tissue transplant

I. Also known as an allograft

J. Skin used to cover a wound that has been obtained from an animal such as a pig

K. An injury resulting from exposure to heat, chemicals, radiation, or electric current; transfer of energy from a source of heat to the human body initiates a sequence of physiological events that in the most severe cases leads to irreversible tissue destruction

L. A burn injury involving only the epidermal layer of the skin; most often results from damage from sunburn, ultraviolet light, a minor flash injury (from a sudden ignition or explosion), or a mild radiation burn associated with cancer treatment

M. Hypovolemic shock resulting from the shift of a massive amount of fluid from the intracellular and intravascular compartments into the interstitium (third spacing)

N. The process of excising a wound to the level of fascia or sequentially removing thin slices of a burn wound to the level of viable tissue

O. A procedure in which a wound is excised to the level of the fascia

P. Another term used to refer to a fascial excision

Q. Condition in which excess pressure constricts the structures within a compartment and reduces circulation to muscles and nerves.

R. Surgical removal of eschar from the torso or extremity to prevent circumferential constriction

S. The surgical, mechanical, or enzymatic removal of all loose tissue, wound debris, and eschar from a wound

T. Skin used for grafting that has been obtained from an animal; also referred to as a heterograft

U. Permanent shortening of connective tissues

V. A burn injury that may be classified as superficial or deep and involves the entire dermis and the papillae of the dermis

FOCUSED STUDY

1. List and describe the phases and activities that take place in the healing of a burn injury.

_____

_____

_____

_____

_____

_____

2. A patient reports to the ambulatory care clinic with a serious sunburn. What interventions should the nurse plan?

_____

_____

_____

_____

_____

3. List and describe the four types of burn injuries.

_____

_____

_____

_____

4. What factors are used to determine the classification of a burn injury?

_____

_____

_____

_____

CASE STUDY

Seventy-four-year-old Viola Baker arrives in the emergency department following a fire in her apartment. She has superficial and superficial partial-thickness burns over 50% of her body, including her face, chest, and arms. Viola was cooking when grease caught fire, catching her clothing on fire as well. There are soot marks around her nostrils, and her eyebrows are singed. She is using a 100% nonrebreather mask and has a pulse oximetry reading of 89%. She is being given normal saline solution by IV in addition to the 5 mg morphine sulfate for pain she was given in the ambulance. Her vital signs are as follows: heart rate 116, blood pressure 104/76, and respiratory rate 35. She opens her eyes to verbal stimuli. Her conversation is confused, but she answers some simple questions and withdraws from pain. The patient's past medical history is significant for osteoporosis, bilateral cataract surgery, and type 2 diabetes mellitus that is controlled with diet and exercise. The patient's family was notified by the apartment manager, and they are on their way to the emergency department.

1. What changes need to be made immediately in the patient's care?

2. To what setting will this patient likely be transferred when she is stable?

3. Why would the patient be intubated and placed on a ventilator?

CARE PLAN CRITICAL-THINKING ACTIVITY

The patient arrives in the emergency department with burns suffered while burning leaves. The initial injury reveals burns to the arms, hands, and facial area. The nurse is planning care for the patient and providing education to the patient and family.

1. What is the greatest concern when this patient first arrives at the emergency room?

2. What unique burn injuries is the patient at risk for developing as a result of the type of burn injury and related situation? What manifestations are noted with this type of burn injury?

3. In assessing respiratory-related injuries, when does the nurse recognize the greatest time for complications as a result of inflammation of the pulmonary system?

REVIEW QUESTIONS

1. The patient, who weighs 68 kg, has sustained second-degree burns over 40% of his body. Which fluid resuscitation is correct according to the Consensus formula?
    1. 10.88 liters of lactated Ringer's solution in 24 hours
    2. 5.44 liters of lactated Ringer's (LR) solution in 8 hours and 10.88 liters of LR over the next 16 hours
    3. 5.44 liters of lactated Ringer's solution in 8 hours and 5.44 liters of D5W over the next 16 hours
    4. 10.88 liters of D5W in 24 hours
2. Which nursing intervention holds the highest priority for a patient with burns to the face and upper respiratory tract?
    1. Elevate the head of the bed to at least 30 degrees.
    2. Administer 6 liters of oxygen via nasal cannula.
    3. Medicate the patient prior to repositioning in bed.
    4. Prevent moving the skin around the burn site.
3. When teaching a community group about radiation burns, which statement best reflects the goals of treatment?
    1. Radiation burns are usually mild and involve only the surface of the skin.
    2. Severe radiation burns are usually caused by industrial accidents.
    3. Radiation burns are much less common than thermal burns.
    4. Promoting wound and body healing are the most important goals of treatment.
4. Which is an appropriate order when caring for a 105-pound patient with a 20% total body surface area burn?
    1. Reduce intake of carbohydrate calories.
    2. Increase intravenous D5W to maintain urine output of 30 mL/hour.
    3. Administer 6 liters of oxygen via nasal cannula without humidification.
    4. Apply support garments beginning on day 5 postgraft.
5. Which is the highest priority when caring for a patient with an electrical burn?
    1. Disconnect the patient from the electrical source.
    2. Ensure that the patient has a cervical collar and is placed on a backboard prior to care.
    3. Monitor for cardiac dysrhythmia.
    4. Provide changes in fluid resuscitation as compared to patients with other types of burns.
6. Which burn wound will require skin grafting in order to heal?
    1. 31.5% superficial radiation burn
    2. 12 mm full-thickness thermal burn
    3. 25% superficial partial-thickness burn to the neck
    4. 18% partial-thickness burn to the lower limbs
7. How is a major burn defined?
    1. 20% total body surface area in adults less than 40 years of age
    2. 5% total body surface area full-thickness burn in adults greater than 40 years of age
    3. a household electrical burn with a cervical spine injury
    4. a burn that caused the oxygen saturation rate to drop below 95%

8. Document on the diagram a burn that involves 22.5% of the patient's body surface area.

Anterior	Totals	Posterior

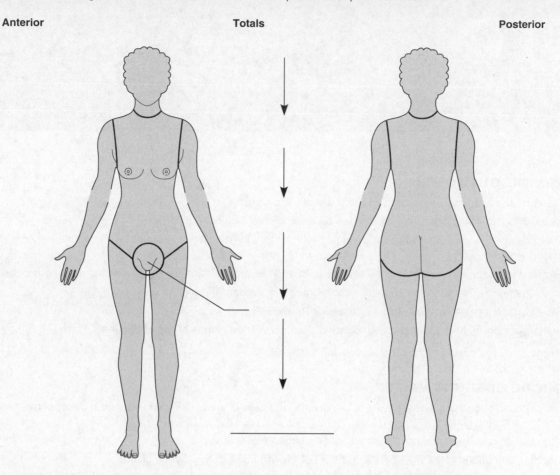

9. Patients with major burns are at risk for many system issues. Which is the highest priority for the nurse caring for a patient with a major burn?
 1. compartment syndrome
 2. hypovolemia
 3. hypothermia
 4. acute renal failure

18

Assessing the Endocrine System

LEARNING OUTCOMES

1. Describe the anatomy and physiology of the endocrine glands.
2. Summarize the functions of the hormones secreted by the endocrine glands.
3. Describe specific topics to consider during a health history interview of the patient with health problems involving endocrine function.
4. Explain techniques for assessing the thyroid gland and the effects of altered function of thyroid hormones.
5. Describe normal variations in endocrine assessment findings for the older adult.
6. Give examples of genetic disorders of the endocrine glands.
7. Identify abnormal findings that may indicate malfunction of the glands of the endocrine system.

CLINICAL COMPETENCIES

1. Conduct and document a health history for patients who have or are at risk for alterations in the structure or function of the endocrine glands.
2. Monitor the results of diagnostic tests and report abnormal findings.
3. Conduct and document a physical assessment of the structure of the thyroid gland.
4. Assess and document the effects of altered endocrine function on other body structures and functions.

TERMS MATCHING

Place the letter of the correct definition in the space next to each term.

1. _____ acromegaly
2. _____ carpal spasm
3. _____ Chvostek's sign
4. _____ dwarfism
5. _____ exophthalmos
6. _____ goiter
7. _____ tetany
8. _____ Trousseau's sign

A. A condition characterized by short stature that is associated with growth hormone deficiency

B. Contraction of the lateral facial muscles in response to tapping the face in front of the ear; caused by decreased blood calcium levels.

C. Protruding eyes, associated with hyperthyroidism

D. An enlarged thyroid gland

E. Contraction of hand and fingers due to hypocalcemia

F. A response that can be elicited by inflating a blood pressure cuff above the antecubital space to a point greater than systolic blood pressure for 2–5 minutes; is indicative of hypocalcemia

G. The continued growth of bone during adulthood from growth hormone hypersecretion

H. Tonic muscle spasms associated with hypocalcemia

FOCUSED STUDY

1. Identify which hormones may be altered in the patient without an adequately functioning anterior pituitary.

   _____

   _____

   _____

2. List several questions the nurse, during the health assessment interview, should ask the patient with a suspected endocrine disorder.

   _____

   _____

   _____

3. The patient's adrenal medulla is hypersecreting catecholamines. Identify what the nurse would expect to find during assessment of the patient.

   _____

   _____

   _____

4. Describe how the nurse should prepare the patient for the water deprivation test.

   _____

   _____

   _____

CASE STUDIES

Case Study 1

Karen Aummert is a 42-year-old female who has come to the physician's office complaining of a decrease in her energy level and feeling sluggish. Her apical heart rate is 56 beats per minute, blood pressure is 98/62, and respiratory rate is 12 per minute. She is recently divorced and is a single parent of a little girl. Answer the following questions based on your knowledge of caring for a patient with an endocrine disorder.

1. Which diagnostic tests might be used to correctly diagnose Ms. Aummert's health problem?

2. Ms. Aummert is diagnosed with hypothyroidism. What can the nurse expect to find during the physical assessment?

3. What are some questions the nurse can ask Ms. Aummert to determine whether she's receiving adequate amounts of sleep and rest?

4. Ms. Aummert states that her 76-year-old mother was recently diagnosed with hypothyroidism. What are some age-related changes that occur in the endocrine system?

Case Study 2

Josh Knight is a 42-year-old male who has been admitted to the hospital with an elevated serum glucose level. The patient collapsed at work and was brought to the hospital via ambulance. Answer the following questions based on your knowledge of caring for a patient with an endocrine disorder.

1. What diagnostic tests may be performed to help the healthcare providers better understand the nature of Mr. Knight's health problem?

2. The nurse questions Mr. Knight regarding his family history of endocrine disorders. Mr. Knight states that his father was diagnosed with diabetes mellitus at the age of 11. Mr. Knight wants to know if other endocrine disorders can be inherited. What is the nurse's best response?

3. Mr. Knight is diagnosed with diabetes mellitus. What are some physical findings associated with this endocrine condition?

SHORT ANSWERS

Glands of the Endocrine System

Fill in the labels for the blanks in the figure. Then compare your answers with Figure 18-1 on page 462 of your textbook.

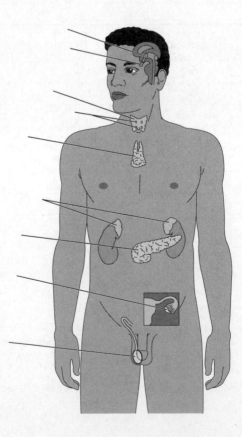

REVIEW QUESTIONS

1. When assessing a patient who is concerned about weight gain, hair loss, and generalized weakness, which assessment is most important?
   1. a focused abdominal assessment
   2. the patient's neck and ability to swallow
   3. the patient's balance and gait
   4. the patient's height and weight

2. The nurse understands that carbohydrate metabolism is most associated with which gland?
   1. pancreas
   2. pituitary
   3. thyroid
   4. parathyroid

3. Epinephrine is produced by which gland?
   1. pancreas
   2. thyroid
   3. adrenal medulla
   4. adrenal cortex

4. A problem with which gland may alter the patient's corticosteroid levels?
   1. thyroid
   2. parathyroid
   3. adrenal cortex
   4. adrenal medulla

5. Which hormone is most responsible for the development of secondary female sexual characteristics?
   1. oxytocin
   2. vasopressin
   3. follicle-stimulating hormone (FSH)
   4. luteinizing hormone (LH)

CHAPTER 19

Nursing Care of Patients with **Endocrine Disorders**

LEARNING OUTCOMES

1. Apply knowledge of normal anatomy, physiology, and assessments of the thyroid, parathyroid, adrenal, and pituitary glands when providing nursing care for patients with endocrine disorders.

2. Compare and contrast the manifestations of disorders that result from hyperfunction and hypofunction of the thyroid, parathyroid, adrenal, and pituitary glands.

3. Explain the nursing implications for medications prescribed to treat disorders of the thyroid and adrenal glands.

4. Provide appropriate nursing care for the patient before and after a subtotal thyroidectomy and an adrenalectomy.

5. Use the nursing process as a framework for providing individualized care to patients with disorders of the thyroid, parathyroid, adrenal, and pituitary glands.

CLINICAL COMPETENCIES

1. Assess the health status of patients with endocrine disorders and monitor, document, and report unexpected or abnormal manifestations.

2. Use assessed data, patient values, clinical expertise, and evidence to determine priority nursing diagnoses and select and implement nursing interventions.

3. Effectively communicate with and function within the interprofessional team to plan and provide patient care.

4. Administer medications knowledgeably and safely.

5. Plan and provide patient and family teaching to promote, restore, and maintain health status.

6. Monitor for respiratory problems and tetany in patients having a thyroidectomy.

7. Adapt individual and cultural values and variations as well as expressed needs and preferences into each patient's plan of care.

8. Evaluate responses to care and use data to revise plan as needed.

TERMS MATCHING

Place the letter of the correct definition in the space next to each term.

1. _____ acromegaly
2. _____ Addisonian crisis
3. _____ Addison's disease
4. _____ Cushing's syndrome
5. _____ diabetes insipidus
6. _____ euthyroid
7. _____ exophthalmos
8. _____ gigantism
9. _____ goiter
10. _____ hyperparathyroidism
11. _____ hypoparathyroidism
12. _____ myxedema
13. _____ myxedema coma
14. _____ proptosis
15. _____ syndrome of inappropriate ADH secretion (SIADH)
16. _____ tetany
17. _____ thyroid crisis or storm
18. _____ thyroidectomy
19. _____ thyroiditis
20. _____ thyrotoxicosis

A. Protrusion of the eyeballs

B. A condition that results from abnormally low PTH levels

C. An enlarged thyroid gland

D. Inflammation of the thyroid gland

E. A life-threatening response to acute adrenal insufficiency

F. A condition also known as hyperthyroidism

G. A condition that results from an increase in the secretion of parathyroid hormone (PTH), which regulates normal serum levels of calcium

H. A severe state of hypothyroidism characterized by edema around the eyes, hands, and feet

I. A disorder resulting from destruction or dysfunction of the adrenal cortex that results in chronic deficiency of cortisol, aldosterone, and adrenal androgens

J. Normal thyroid function

K. Forward displacement in the eye as associated with Graves' disease

L. A condition that occurs when GH hypersecretion begins before puberty and the closure of the epiphyseal plates

M. Surgical removal of all or part of the thyroid gland

N. A chronic disorder caused by excessive amounts of circulating cortisol

O. An extreme state of hyperthyroidism

P. A condition characterized by abnormally high levels of ADH

Q. A life-threatening complication of long-standing, untreated hypothyroidism, characterized by severe metabolic disorders (hyponatremia, hypoglycemia, lactic acidosis), hypothermia, cardiovascular collapse, impaired cognition, and coma

R. Meaning literally "enlarged extremities," this is a condition resulting from excessive growth hormone secretion during adulthood

S. Tonic muscular spasms; a sign of hypocalcemia

T. A condition that is the result of ADH insufficiency

FOCUSED STUDY

1. Discuss manifestations and treatment of hyperthyroidism.

   a. Manifestations

   _____

   _____

   b. Treatment

   _____

   _____

2. Discuss the manifestations of hypothyroidism.

_____

_____

_____

_____

3. Discuss the treatment for Cushing's syndrome.

_____

_____

_____

_____

4. Compare and contrast gigantism and acromegaly.

_____

_____

_____

_____

5. Discuss the differences between the clinical manifestations associated with diabetes insipidus and syndrome of inappropriate antidiuretic hormone (SIADH) secretion.

_____

_____

_____

_____

CASE STUDY

Judy Moss is a 43-year-old White female who was recently diagnosed with Addison's disease. Answer the following questions based on your knowledge of caring for patients with endocrine disorders.

1. How should the nurse explain Addison's disease to Ms. Moss?

2. What manifestations should the nurse look for during the assessment of Ms. Moss?

3. What skin changes should the nurse expect Ms. Moss to experience?

4. What diagnostic testing procedures may have been used to diagnose Ms. Moss's condition?

5. What medications can be used to treat Ms. Moss?

6. What should the nurse include when educating Ms. Moss about self-care techniques?

SHORT ANSWERS

Fill in the missing pieces regarding the pathophysiology of Cushing's syndrome.

Manifestations	Pathophysiology
Weight gain, abdominal fat deposits, fat pads on the upper back ("buffalo hump"), and a round face ("moon face")	
Muscle weakness and wasting, especially in the extremities	
Thinning of skin, abdominal striae, easy bruising, poor wound healing	
Osteoporosis, compression fractures of the vertebrae, and rib fractures	
Increased susceptability to infections	
Hypertension, hypokalemia, and hypernatremia	
Hyperglycemia, polyuria, and polydipsia	
Increased risk for deep vein thrombosis	
Increased risk of gastric ulcers	
Hirsutism, acne, and menstrual irregularities	
Emotional instability	

REVIEW QUESTIONS

1. The patient has been diagnosed with hyperthyroidism. As the nurse reviewing the patient's chart, which finding would you consider unexpected?
   1. increased appetite
   2. insomnia
   3. increased sweating
   4. constipation
2. The patient has been diagnosed with thyroid storm. Identify the inappropriate nursing intervention to use with this patient.
   1. Replace fluids.
   2. Reduce body temperature by administering aspirin.
   3. Apply oxygen.
   4. Replace electrolytes.
3. The patient has hyperthyroidism. Which behavior demonstrates that education has been adequate?
   1. The patient participates in almost continuous activity.
   2. The patient practices stress-reduction techniques.
   3. The patient weighs herself weekly.
   4. The patient restricts carbohydrates and protein in her diet.
4. The nurse will administer which medication to the patient with hypothyroidism to increase thyroid hormone level?
   1. phenytoin
   2. levothyroxine sodium
   3. lithium
   4. propranolol

5. The nurse has provided education for the patient regarding Hashimoto's thyroiditis. Which statement by the patient indicates the need for further education?
   1. "It is more common in men."
   2. "It is an autoimmune disorder."
   3. "It causes a goiter to form."
   4. "It has a familial link."

6. The nurse understands that which patient population is less likely to develop hypercortisolism?
   1. women between the ages of 30 and 50
   2. males who are teenagers
   3. patients prescribed long-term steroids
   4. patients undergoing chemotherapy

7. Identify the behavior that demonstrates the patient's understanding of the education regarding Cushing's syndrome.
   1. The patient refuses to discuss his or her body changes with professionals.
   2. The patient decreases intake of vitamins A and C in his or her diet.
   3. The patient restricts fluids.
   4. The patient uses dim lighting.

8. Patients experience clinical manifestations associated with Addison's disease after what percent of adrenal gland function is lost?
   1. 40%
   2. 50%
   3. 70%
   4. 90%

Nursing Care of Patients with Diabetes Mellitus

LEARNING OUTCOMES

1. Describe the prevalence and incidence of diabetes mellitus (DM).
2. Explain the pathophysiology, risk factors, manifestations, and complications of type 1 and type 2 DM.
3. Provide the rationale for diagnostic tests used for screening, diagnosis, and monitoring of DM.
4. Discuss the nursing implications for insulin and oral hypoglycemic agents used to treat patients with DM.
5. Discuss best practices of self-care management of DM related to diet planning, sick day management, and exercise.
6. Compare and contrast the manifestations of hypoglycemia, diabetic ketoacidosis (DKA), and hyperosmolar hyperglycemic state (HHS).

CLINICAL COMPETENCIES

1. Assess blood glucose levels and patterns of hyper- and hypoglycemia in patients with DM.
2. Use assessed data, patient values, clinical expertise, and evidence to determine priority nursing diagnoses and select and implement individualized nursing interventions.
3. Administer oral and injectable medications used to treat DM knowledgeably and safely.
4. Provide individualized care to patients with hypoglycemia, diabetic ketoacidosis, and hyperosmolar hyperglycemic state.
5. Effectively communicate with and function within the interprofessional team to plan and provide patient care.
6. Provide appropriate teaching to facilitate self-monitoring of blood glucose, administration of oral and injectable hypoglycemic medications, diabetic diet, appropriate exercise, and effective foot care.
7. Adapt individual and cultural values and variations as well as expressed needs and preferences into the plan of care for patients with DM.
8. Revise the plan of care as needed to provide effective interventions to promote, maintain, or restore normal glucose levels.

TERMS MATCHING

Place the letter of the correct definition in the space next to each term.

1. _____ diabetes mellitus (DM)

2. _____ diabetic ketoacidosis (DKA)

3. _____ gastroparesis

4. _____ gluconeogenesis

5. _____ glucosuria

6. _____ glycogenolysis

7. _____ hyperglycemia

8. _____ hyperosmolar hyperglycemic state (HHS)

9. _____ hypoglycemia

10. _____ ketosis

11. _____ metabolic syndrome

12. _____ polydipsia

13. _____ polyphagia

14. _____ polyuria

15. _____ positive urine glucose

16. _____ prediabetes

17. _____ urine ketone tests

A. Slowed gastrointestinal motility, which causes early satiety

B. Excessive glucose in urine

C. The breakdown of liver glycogen to glucose

D. Eating more food in response to energy decreases in type I diabetes

E. Blood sugar is higher than normal but not yet high enough to be classified as type 2 diabetes

F. An accumulation of ketone bodies produced during the oxidation of fatty acids

G. The formation of glucose from fats and proteins

H. A cluster of manifestations associated with type 2 DM. Includes hypertension, visceral obesity, low HDL, high triglycerides, elevated C-reactive protein and fasting glucose >110 mg/dL

I. An elevated blood glucose level

J. Drinking large amounts of fluid

K. Group of chronic disorders of the endocrine pancreas, all categorized under a broad diagnostic label. The condition is characterized by inappropriate hyperglycemia caused by a relative or absolute deficiency of insulin or by a cellular resistance to the action of insulin

L. A metabolic disorder characterized by plasma osmolarity of 340 mOsm/L or greater (the normal range is 280–300 mOsm/L), greatly elevated blood glucose levels (over 600 mg/dL and often 1,000–2,000 mg/dL), and altered levels of consciousness

M. Low blood glucose levels

N. Production of large amounts of urine

O. Presence of glucose found in urine; however, not reliable as glucose does not appear in the urine below the renal threshold of 180 mg/dL

P. A form of metabolic acidosis induced by stress in a person with type 1 diabetes

Q. Used to determine whether fats are being metabolized for energy, marking the beginning of diabetic ketoacidosis

FOCUSED STUDY

1. Describe the differences between type 1 and type 2 diabetes.

_____

_____

_____

_____

_____

2. What diagnostic tests are used to manage diabetes?

_____

_____

_____

_____

_____

3. Describe the different types of insulin preparations.

_____

_____

_____

_____

_____

4. Explain the cause of diabetic ketoacidosis (DKA) and its treatment.

_____

_____

_____

_____

_____

5. Discuss the primary treatment modalities that are used to manage the patient with hyperosmolar hyperglycemic state.

_____

_____

_____

_____

_____

CASE STUDY

Jack Brown is a 56-year-old male who was recently diagnosed with diabetes. He has spent the past 3 days on the unit with a diagnosis of hypoglycemia secondary to diabetes. He is being discharged with prescriptions for an oral hypoglycemic. Answer the following questions based on your knowledge of caring for patients with diabetes.

1. With what type of diabetes would Mr. Brown be diagnosed? Why?

2. How do oral hypoglycemics regulate blood sugar?

3. What modifications will Mr. Brown need to make to his diet?

4. How should Mr. Brown be taught to manage an episode of hypoglycemia?

5. Mr. Brown asks about the types of complications that may accompany his condition. What disorders are linked to diabetes mellitus?

SHORT ANSWERS

Fill in the table.

Drug Name	Classification	Onset (hrs)	Peak (hrs)	Duration (hrs)
Lispro				
Humulin R®				
Humulin N®				
Levemir				
Lantus®				

REVIEW QUESTIONS

1. The nurse understands which statement to be true about type 2 diabetes mellitus?
   1. Its onset begins most often in childhood.
   2. It is the nonketonic form of diabetes.
   3. It can be triggered by a viral infection.
   4. An exogenous source of insulin is required.

2. What is the normal fasting glucose level?
   1. 40 mg/dL
   2. 60 mg/dL
   3. 100 mg/dL
   4. 200 mg/dL

3. Which syringe is not available for administering insulin?
   1. 0.3 mL (30 U)
   2. 0.5 mL (50 U)
   3. 1.0 mL (100 U)
   4. 1.5 mL (150 U)

4. Identify the incorrect method of insulin injection.
   1. Inject the needle at a 90-degree angle.
   2. Massage the site after administering the injection.
   3. Rotate sites of injection.
   4. Do not inject insulin into an area that will be exercised.

5. The dawn phenomenon is a rise in blood glucose between what hours?
   1. 12 AM–2 AM
   2. 3 AM–8 AM
   3. 4 AM–8 AM
   4. 6 AM–9 AM

6. Which behavior indicates that the patient is following instructions for proper foot care?
   1. The patient inspects the feet monthly for changes.
   2. The patient wears tight-fitting shoes to facilitate circulation.
   3. The patient keeps the feet in a dependent position the majority of the day.
   4. After bathing the feet, the patient pats the foot dry and dries the areas between the toes well.

Assessing the Gastrointestinal System

LEARNING OUTCOMES

1. Discuss the function of nutrients absorbed in the gastrointestinal (GI) system.
2. Describe the anatomy, physiology, and functions of the GI system and the accessory digestive organs.
3. Identify focused topics to consider during a health history interview of the patient with GI disorders.
4. Explain techniques used for assessing nutritional status and GI function.
5. Describe normal variations in GI assessment findings for the older adult.
6. Identify abnormal findings that may indicate alterations in GI function.
7. Give examples of common genetic disorders of the GI system.

CLINICAL COMPETENCIES

1. Conduct and document a health history for patients who have or are at risk for alterations in GI function, eliciting patient values, preferences, and expressed needs as part of the interview.
2. Conduct and document a physical assessment of nutritional status and the GI system, demonstrating sensitivity and respect for dietary habits related to culture and individual belief systems.
3. Provide supportive nursing care for patients undergoing invasive diagnostic procedures.
4. Monitor the results of diagnostic tests and report abnormal findings.

TERMS MATCHING

Place the letter of the correct definition in the space next to each term.

1. _____ bile

2. _____ borborygmus

3. _____ bruit

4. _____ cheilosis

5. _____ dietary reference intakes (DRIs)

6. _____ flatus

7. _____ gingivitis

8. _____ glossitis

9. _____ hernia

10. _____ leukoplakia

11. _____ melena

12. _____ nutrition

13. _____ ostomy

14. _____ steatorrhea

15. _____ striae

16. _____ tolerable upper intake level

17. _____ Valsalva's maneuver

A. Cracks at corners of the mouth seen in vitamin B-complex deficiencies, especially riboflavin

B. Intestinal gas

C. Formation of white patches or spots on the mucous membranes or tongue; these lesions may become malignant

D. The process by which the body, via the gastrointestinal system and the accessory digestive organs, ingests, absorbs, transports, uses, and eliminates nutrients in food

E. The presence of excessive loud and hyperactive bowel sounds; auscultated in patients with diarrhea or bowel obstructions

F. Performed by closing the glottis and contracting the diaphragm and abdominal muscles to increase intra-abdominal pressure

G. Black, tarry stool that contains old, digested blood

H. Greasy, frothy, yellow stools resulting from excess fat in the feces

I. A defect in the abdominal wall that allows abdominal contents to protrude outward

J. Swollen, red gums that bleed easily

K. A surgical opening into a patient's bowel

L. A smooth, bright red tongue

M. An adventitious sound heard during auscultation; of venous or arterial origin

N. The maximum level of daily nutrient intake that is likely to pose no risk of adverse effects

O. The recommended intakes of nutrients (vitamins & elements) as labeled by the National Academy of Sciences

P. A line above or below tissue that differs in color and texture from surrounding tissue

Q. A greenish, watery solution containing bile salts, cholesterol, bilirubin, electrolytes, water, and phospholipids

FOCUSED STUDY

1. Locate and label the major digestive and accessory digestive organs in the diagram. Then compare your answers with Figure 21-1 on page 539 of your textbook.

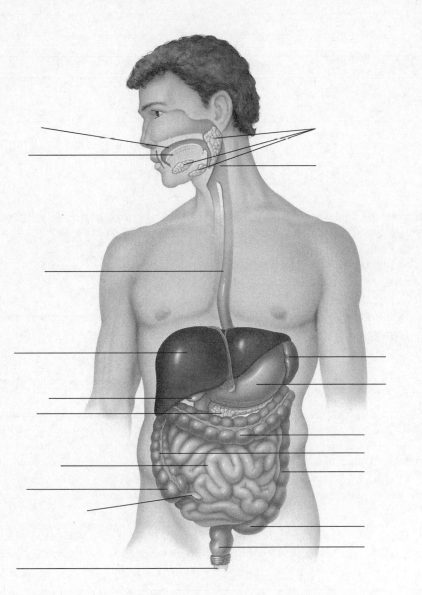

2. Describe the following nutrient categories and provide an example of each.

a. Carbohydrates

_____

_____

b. Proteins

_____

_____

c. Fats

_____

_____

3. Describe how the autonomic nervous system (parasympathetic and sympathetic) influences the production of gastric secretions.

_____

_____

_____

_____

_____

4. Calculate your body mass index.

_____

CASE STUDIES

Case Study 1

During a community health screening, a 36-year-old patient states that he has been experiencing epigastric pain three to five times per week. Answer the following questions based on your knowledge of the digestive system.

1. What questions should the nurse ask this patient?

2. Epigastric pain can be associated with what disorders?

3. The patient has been scheduled for an esophagogastroduodenoscopy. What are the nurse's responsibilities regarding caring for this patient?

Case Study 2

Jerry Parsons is an 86-year-old male who is being seen in the physician's office. He is complaining of constipation. Answer the following based on your knowledge of the digestive system.

1. Mr. Parsons states, "It seems as though my problems with constipation have gotten worse as I have gotten older." How should the nurse respond?

2. What could result from frequent bouts of constipation?

3. What radiographic study may be performed to assess Mr. Parsons's rectum and colon?

SHORT ANSWERS

The nurse is assessing a patient who is experiencing malnutrition. Complete the table by identifying the expected assessment findings.

Body System	Assessment Findings
Nails	
Hair	
Skin	
Eyes	
Nervous system	
Musculoskeletal system	
Cardiovascular system	
GI system	

REVIEW QUESTIONS

1. When obtaining a medical history from a patient, the nurse learns that all of his duodenum and several feet of small intestine were removed. What concerns should the nurse have regarding this patient's nutritional status related to the location of the removal?
   1. malabsorption
   2. loose stools and potential for dehydration
   3. poor production of vitamin D
   4. inadequate bile production

2. During the male patient's assessment, which finding is indicative that he is experiencing malnutrition?
   1. Triceps skin fold thickness is 13.0 mm.
   2. Midarm muscle circumference is 300 mm.
   3. Body mass index (BMI) is 18.
   4. Midarm circumference (MAC) is 301 mm.

3. When the nurse percusses the lower border of the liver, the dullness ends at the costal margin. What does the nurse know about this finding?
   1. It is indicative of cirrhosis.
   2. It is indicative of venous congestion of the liver.
   3. It is a normal finding.
   4. It is indicative of hepatitis.

4. Which statement regarding the assessment of bowel sounds is accurate?
   1. Bowel sounds are most active in the upper left quadrant.
   2. If bowel sounds are absent in each quadrant, it may take up to 20 minutes to assess.
   3. Bowel sounds should be heard within the first 5 seconds of auscultation.
   4. Bowel sounds should sound high pitched, tinkling, or rushing.

5. A patient describes painful vertical fissures on the tongue. With what are these most likely associated?
   1. riboflavin deficiency
   2. dehydration
   3. folic acid deficiency
   4. antibiotic use

6. What is the first step of assessing the abdomen?
   1. auscultate
   2. inspect
   3. percuss
   4. palpate

7. While assessing the anus and rectum, the advanced practice nurse's initial action is to slowly insert a gloved finger into the patient's anus and point it toward the
   1. descending colon.
   2. umbilicus.
   3. right lung.
   4. liver.

CHAPTER 22

Nursing Care of Patients with **Nutritional Disorders**

LEARNING OUTCOMES

1. Describe the pathophysiology and clinical manifestations of common nutritional disorders.
2. Identify risk factors for nutritional disorders and nursing measures to reduce those risks.
3. Identify causes, effects, and complications of nutritional disorders on general patient health status.
4. Describe effective interprofessional care for patients with nutritional disorders.
5. Develop strategies to promote nutrition for patient populations.

CLINICAL COMPETENCIES

1. Assess and monitor the health status of patients with nutritional disorders, recognizing and reporting unexpected manifestations or responses to treatment.
2. Use technology and information management tools to provide preventive interventions and health teaching for patients and populations at risk for developing complications resulting from nutritional disorders.
3. Using assessment data, research, and current standards of practice, plan and implement evidence-based nursing care for patients with nutritional disorders.
4. Administer medications and enteral and parenteral nutrition knowledgeably and safely.
5. Collaborate and coordinate with the patient and other members of the interprofessional care team to prioritize and implement care.
6. Incorporate cultural values and customs and personal preferences into the plan of care for patients with nutritional disorders.
7. Use holistic data to plan and provide care and to evaluate care and responses to interventions focused on health teaching and health coaching.

TERMS MATCHING

Place the letter of the correct definition in the space next to each term.

1. _____ anorexia nervosa
2. _____ bariatrics
3. _____ basal metabolic rate (BMR)
4. _____ binge-eating disorder
5. _____ body mass index (BMI)
6. _____ bulimia nervosa
7. _____ catabolism
8. _____ enteral nutrition
9. _____ lower body obesity
10. _____ malnutrition
11. _____ metabolic syndrome
12. _____ nutrients
13. _____ obesity
14. _____ parenteral nutrition (PN)
15. _____ protein-calorie malnutrition (PCM)
16. _____ sarcopenic obesity
17. _____ starvation
18. _____ triglycerides
19. _____ upper body obesity
20. _____ very-low-calorie diets (VLCDs)

A. An eating disorder characterized by recurring episodes of binge eating followed by purge behaviors
B. Inadequate nutrient intake to meet body needs
C. Molecules of glycerol with fatty acids used to transport and store fats in body tissues
D. An excess of adipose tissue and a BMI greater than 30 kg/m^2
E. Deficient protein and calories to meet metabolic needs
F. Diet programs that offer a protein-sparing modified fast (800 kcal/day or less) under close medical supervision
G. An eating disorder characterized by a body weight less than 85% of expected for age and height, and intense fear of gaining weight or of losing control over food intake
H. The process of muscle loss combined with increased body fat as people age, leading to a loss of function and reduced quality of life
I. Central obesity
J. Peripheral obesity
K. A cluster of manifestations associated with type 2 DM. Includes hypertension, visceral obesity, low HDL, high triglycerides, elevated C-reactive protein and fasting glucose > 110 mg/dL
L. Test to measure the energy used when the body is at rest; rarely used due to the availability of more accurate thyroid tests
M. Biochemical process involving the breakdown of complex structures into simpler forms
N. Inadequate dietary intake
O. Substances found in food that are used by the body to promote growth, maintenance, and repair
P. A nutritional disorder that is characterized by eating an excessive amount of food during a defined period of time
Q. Tube feeding
R. An indirect measure of the amount of body fat
S. The healthcare science that focuses on patients who are extremely obese
T. The intravenous administration of amino acids, often with added carbohydrates, fats, electrolytes, vitamins, and minerals

FOCUSED STUDY

1. Define obesity and explain its health concerns.

_____

2. Describe the forms of bariatric procedures performed in the United States.

_____
_____
_____
_____

3. Describe the manifestations that patients with malnutrition will experience.

_____
_____
_____
_____
_____

4. Explain the difference between anorexia nervosa and bulimia nervosa.

_____
_____
_____
_____

CASE STUDY

Barbara Spencer is a 50-year-old woman who has been diagnosed with binge-eating disorder. She has been referred to the mental health unit for counseling. Answer the following questions based on your knowledge of caring for patients with a binge-eating disorder.

1. What psychosocial factors may have contributed to Ms. Spencer's eating disorder?

2. What diagnostic studies may be ordered to assess Ms. Spencer's nutritional status?

3. What treatments are instituted for patients with a binge-eating disorder?

4. What role can Ms. Spencer's family play in assisting her to be successful with her treatment regimen?

SHORT ANSWERS

Fill in the table regarding nutritional deficiencies. Identify assessment data related to each nutritional deficiency listed.

Deficiency	Assessment Data
Calorie	
Protein	
Vitamin A	
Thiamine	
Riboflavin	
Vitamin C	
Iron	

REVIEW QUESTIONS

1. The nurse understands that a patient with a BMI of greater than _____ kg/m^2 has obesity.
   1. 20
   2. 23
   3. 27
   4. 30

2. What is the most important factor that contributes to obesity?
   1. physical inactivity
   2. genetics
   3. ethnicity
   4. increased access to inexpensive foods

3. Which is not a manifestation of metabolic syndrome?
   1. increased waist circumference
   2. high HDL cholesterol
   3. hypertension
   4. an increase in fasting blood glucose

4. The patient reports fecal urgency. The nurse recognizes this as a side effect of which medication?
   1. Belviq® (lorcaserin)
   2. Tenuate® (diethylproprion)
   3. Prozac® (fluoxetine)
   4. Xenical® (orlistat)

5. The patient reports a history of stomach reduction surgery that can be adjusted by changing the amount of saline injected. The nurse knows that the patient underwent which of the following procedures?
   1. biliopancreatic diversion
   2. Roux-en-Y gastric bypass
   3. adjustable gastric banding
   4. vertical banded gastroplasty

6. Which nursing intervention is not appropriate for a patient who needs to reduce her weight?
   1. Assist the patient to identify cues to eating.
   2. Establish a weight loss goal of 3–4 pounds per week.
   3. Assist the patient to develop a well-balanced food menu.
   4. Monitor laboratory values.

7. The patient presents with malnutrition. The nurse should assess the patient for which manifestation?
   1. oily, limp hair
   2. weight loss of greater than 10% of usual weight
   3. inability to eat for more than 2 days
   4. affluent lifestyle

8. Which finding requires an immediate intervention when the nurse is monitoring the patient's parenteral nutrition?
   1. The nurse finds that the nutrition is being infused through a central line.
   2. The solution is being administered by gravity.
   3. The intravenous fluid hanging contains 10% dextrose.
   4. The parenteral solution is found to be mixed with intralipids.

9. Dumping syndrome occurs with diets that are high in what nutrient?
   1. fiber
   2. protein
   3. simple carbohydrates
   4. fat

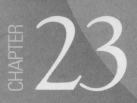

CHAPTER 23

Nursing Care of Patients with **Upper Gastrointestinal Disorders**

LEARNING OUTCOMES

1. Describe the pathophysiology of common disorders of the mouth, esophagus, and stomach.
2. Distinguish manifestations and diagnostic test results and correlate with the pathophysiologic processes involved in upper gastrointestinal disorders.
3. Explain interprofessional care for patients with upper gastrointestinal disorders.
4. Describe the role of the nurse in interprofessional care of patients with upper gastrointestinal disorders.

CLINICAL COMPETENCIES

1. Assess the health status of patients with upper gastrointestinal disorders.
2. Monitor, identify, document, and report significant manifestations of upper gastrointestinal disorders and their complications.
3. Plan patient-centered nursing care using evidence-based practice guidelines, research, and, as appropriate, health information technology.
4. Determine priority nursing diagnoses, problems, and interventions based on assessed data.
5. Administer medications and prescribed care knowledgeably and safely.
6. Integrate and coordinate interprofessional care into the plan of care.
7. Construct and revise individualized plans of care considering the culture and values of the patient.
8. Plan and provide patient and family teaching to promote, maintain, and restore health.

TERMS MATCHING

Place the letter of the correct definition in the space next to each term.

1. _____ achalasia

2. _____ anorexia

3. _____ Curling's ulcers

4. _____ Cushing's ulcers

5. _____ dumping syndrome

6. _____ dysphagia

7. _____ erosive (stress-induced) gastritis

8. _____ gastric mucosal barrier

9. _____ gastritis

10. _____ gastroesophageal reflux

11. _____ hematemesis

12. _____ hematochezia

13. _____ melena

14. _____ nausea

15. _____ occult bleeding

16. _____ partial gastrectomy

17. _____ peptic ulcer disease (PUD)

18. _____ peptic ulcers

19. _____ steatorrhea

20. _____ stomatitis

21. _____ total gastrectomy

22. _____ ulcer

23. _____ vomiting

24. _____ Zollinger-Ellison syndrome

A. Blood in the vomit

B. The forceful expulsion of the contents of the upper gastrointestinal tract resulting from contraction of muscles in the gut and abdominal wall

C. A chronic disease that occurs as a result of a break in the mucous lining of the gastrointestinal tract where it comes in contact with gastric secretions

D. Absence of peristalsis of the esophagus and high gastroesophageal sphincter pressure resulting in dilation and loss of tone in the esophagus

E. Can occur in any area of the gastrointestinal tract exposed to acid-pepsin secretions, including the esophagus, stomach, and duodenum

F. Loss of appetite

G. Greasy, frothy, yellow stools resulting from excess fat in the feces

H. Inflammation of the stomach lining that results from irritation of the gastric mucosa

I. A lesion of the skin or mucous membranes

J. The backward flowing of gastric contents into the esophagus

K. Blood in the stool

L. Complication of partial gastrectomy characterized by nausea, weakness, sweating, palpitation, syncope, sensation of warmth, and occasionally diarrhea

M. Black, tarry stool

N. Stress ulcers occurring as sequelae of head injury or central nervous system surgery

O. The surgical removal of the entire stomach

P. Protects the stomach from hydrochloric acid and pepsin

Q. A term used to describe inflammation and ulcers of the oral mucosa

R. A type of peptic ulcer disease that is caused by a gastrinoma, or a gastrin-secreting tumor of the pancreas, stomach, or intestines

S. The surgical removal of a portion of the stomach

T. Inflammation and superficial erosions of the gastric mucosa that may occur as a complication of other life-threatening conditions such as shock, severe trauma, major surgery, sepsis, burns, or head injury

U. Acute ulcerations of the stomach or duodenum that form following a burn injury

V. Difficult or painful swallowing

W. A vague, unpleasant sensation of sickness or queasiness

X. Bleeding that is unnoticed by the patient

FOCUSED STUDY

1. List several risk factors for developing stomatitis.

_____

_____

_____

_____

2. Discuss the clinical manifestations that can be found in the patient with oral cancer.

_____

_____

_____

_____

3. Discuss the nursing interventions that should be provided for the patient with a disturbed sleep pattern due to peptic ulcer disease.

_____

_____

_____

_____

4. Describe interprofessional care that can be provided for the patient with acute or chronic gastritis. Discuss the differences between how acute and chronic gastritis are typically diagnosed.

_____

_____

_____

CASE STUDY

Kevin Hess is a 40-year-old male who has been diagnosed with a duodenal ulcer. He states that he has smoked approximately two packs of cigarettes per day since he was 17 years old. He admits to using ibuprofen in large amounts to ease chronic pain in his right knee. Answer the following questions based on your knowledge of caring for patients with peptic ulcer disease.

1. What role does Mr. Hess's age, smoking history, and ibuprofen use play in his peptic ulcer disease?

2. Why might Mr. Hess be screened for *H. pylori* infection?

3. As the nurse assesses Mr. Hess, what are some expected findings regarding his description of symptoms?

4. Describe the clinical manifestations Mr. Hess may experience if he develops the most lethal complication of peptic ulcer disease.

5. Mr. Hess's physician has prescribed lansoprazole (Prevacid®). How should the nurse educate Mr. Hess regarding how he should take this medication?

6. During the nurse's assessment of Mr. Hess, he begins to hemorrhage. What are some clinical manifestations the nurse may discover with this condition?

7. What are several nursing concerns to consider when developing Mr. Hess's plan of care?

CARE PLAN CRITICAL-THINKING ACTIVITY

1. Mr. Chavez, a patient diagnosed with oral cancer, states that he quit smoking, but the nurse sees a pack of cigarettes in his shirt pocket and he smells of smoke. What should the nurse do?

2. What techniques can be used to assist Mr. Chavez to communicate during the immediate postoperative period?

3. What behaviors will demonstrate that Mr. Chavez's anxiety has lessened about his speech?

SHORT ANSWERS

Fill in the table. Identify the pathophysiology associated with each clinical manifestation of GERD.

Manifestation	Pathophysiology
Heartburn Chest pain Regurgitation Belching	
Dysphagia	
Pain after eating	
Chronic cough Hoarseness Laryngitis, pharyngitis	

REVIEW QUESTIONS

1. The patient has been diagnosed with oral cancer. Which place in the mouth is an unexpected site for oral cancer to develop?
   1. tongue
   2. upper lip
   3. lower lip
   4. floor of the mouth

2. The nurse expects that the patient will be unable to communicate verbally following oral surgery. Which technique would help the nurse communicate most effectively with the patient after surgery?
   1. Have the patient record all questions preoperatively on a tape recorder.
   2. Require that a spokesperson be available at the patient's bedside at all times.
   3. Place a writing tablet and pens next to the bed.
   4. Provide the patient with the cell phone numbers of the nursing staff's unit.

3. The patient has been diagnosed with gastroesophageal reflux disease. Which order is unexpected by the nurse?
   1. Prepare the patient for a barium enema.
   2. Prepare the patient for 24-hour ambulatory pH monitoring.
   3. Prepare the patient for a barium swallow.
   4. Obtain consent for an upper gastrointestinal endoscopy.

4. Adenocarcinoma is one of two forms of esophageal cancer. What is the other form of esophageal cancer?
   1. squamous cell
   2. basal cell
   3. epithelial cell
   4. stratus cell

5. The patient has been vomiting for the last 6 days and has developed the following problems. Which finding would be an unexpected complication of vomiting?
   1. hyperkalemia
   2. metabolic acidosis
   3. aspiration
   4. tears of the esophagus

6. To help relieve nausea and vomiting, the nurse could suggest using which aromatic root?
   1. anise
   2. catmint
   3. sage
   4. ginger

7. Which patient statement reflects an adequate understanding of how to prevent dumping syndrome?
   1. "I eat three large meals a day."
   2. "I do not drink liquids with my meals."
   3. "I have decreased the amount of protein in my diet."
   4. "I have increased the amount of sugar in my diet."

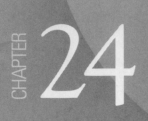

CHAPTER 24

Nursing Care of Patients with **Bowel Disorders**

LEARNING OUTCOMES

1. Compare and contrast the causes, pathophysiology, manifestations, interprofessional care, and nursing care of patients with disorders of bowel motility.

2. Explain the pathophysiology, manifestations, complications, interprofessional care, and nursing care of patients with acute or chronic inflammatory bowel disorders, and structural and obstructive bowel disorders.

3. Discuss the purposes, nursing implications, and health education for the patient and family related to medications used to treat bowel disorders.

4. Explain the rationale for using selected diets, including those for diarrhea and constipation and low-residue, gluten-free, and high-fiber diets.

5. Describe selected surgical procedures of the bowel, including colectomy, colostomy, ileostomy, and perianal surgery.

CLINICAL COMPETENCIES

1. Assess the functional status of patients with bowel disorders, and recognize, document, and report unexpected or abnormal findings.

2. Use assessment data to determine priority nursing diagnoses, identify and implement patient-centered evidence-based nursing interventions, and revise the plan of care for patients with bowel disorders.

3. Integrate interprofessional care and administer medications knowledgeably and safely for patients with bowel disorders.

4. Provide skilled care to patients having bowel surgery, an ostomy, or perianal surgery.

5. Provide culturally appropriate teaching to promote nutrition, prevent acute and chronic bowel disorders, encourage screening, and facilitate continuity of care related to bowel disorders.

TERMS MATCHING

Place the letter of the correct definition in the space next to each term.

1. _____ borborygmi
2. _____ colectomy
3. _____ colostomy
4. _____ constipation
5. _____ diarrhea
6. _____ hematochezia
7. _____ ileostomy
8. _____ inflammatory bowel disease (IBD)
9. _____ malabsorption
10. _____ paralytic ileus
11. _____ peritonitis
12. _____ steatorrhea
13. _____ stoma

A. Greasy, frothy, yellow stools resulting from excess fat in the feces
B. The surgical creation of an opening from the large bowel on the abdominal wall
C. An ostomy made in the ileum of the small intestine
D. A condition in which the intestinal mucosa ineffectively absorbs nutrients, resulting in their excretion in the stool
E. Inflammation of the peritoneum; a serious complication of many acute abdominal disorders
F. Excessively loud, hyperactive bowel sounds
G. Stools that are obviously bloody
H. A group of disorders that includes Crohn's disease and ulcerative colitis; these conditions cause inflammation in the digestive tract
I. The opening on the surface of the wall of abdomen that is created when an ostomy is created
J. The surgical resection and removal of the colon
K. The impaired propulsion or forward movement of bowel contents
L. An increase in the frequency, volume, and fluid content of the stool; the water content of feces is increased
M. Two or fewer bowel movements weekly or difficulty passing stools

FOCUSED STUDY

1. List five risk factors that may contribute to the development of constipation.

_____
_____
_____

2. Describe the clinical manifestations that may be found in a patient who has been diagnosed with peritonitis. Describe the clinical manifestations that may found in a patient who develops a systemic infection due to peritonitis.

_____
_____
_____
_____

3. Describe the different ways diverticular disease can be treated.

_____
_____
_____

4. List the three different types of polyps. Explain how polyps are usually diagnosed.

_____
_____

CASE STUDY

Lynn Bowman is a 16-year-old female who comes into the emergency room with complaints of right lower quadrant pain, nausea, vomiting, and a fever of 101°F. With palpation, she exhibits rebound tenderness at McBurney's point. She is diagnosed with appendicitis. Answer the following questions based on your knowledge of caring for patients with appendicitis.

1. Where is McBurney's point located?

2. What are possible complications of untreated appendicitis?

3. What diagnostic studies may be used to diagnose appendicitis?

4. Prior to an appendectomy, what medications may be ordered for Ms. Bowman?

5. Ms. Bowman undergoes an appendectomy. What should the nurse's postoperative teaching include?

6. What two nursing concerns might the nurse have in regard to Ms. Bowman's plan of care following surgery?

SHORT ANSWERS

Fill in the table. Note whether the laboratory value will be "increased," "decreased," or "within normal limits" when the patient has been experiencing severe diarrhea.

Test	Normal Value	Change with Significant Diarrhea
Serum osmolality	280–300 mOsm/kg	
Serum potassium	3.5–5.3 mEq/L	
Serum sodium	135–145 mEq/L	
Serum chloride	95–105 mEq/L	
Blood gases		
pH	Arterial: 7.35–7.45	
PCO_2	Arterial: 35–45 mmHg	
Bicarbonate	24–28 mEq/L	
Hematocrit	Males: 40%–54%	
	Females: 36%–46%	
Urine specific gravity	1.005–1.030	

REVIEW QUESTIONS

1. What dietary instruction should the nurse give the patient about managing acute diarrhea?

    1. Eat foods high in fiber.

    2. Eat small, frequent meals.

    3. Avoid drinking electrolyte solutions such as Gatorade®.

    4. Increase the intake of milk products.

2. Which statement demonstrates that the patient understands teaching about managing constipation?

    1. "I should limit my fluid intake."

    2. "I should avoid bran and prunes."

    3. "I should participate in a daily form of exercise."

    4. "I should avoid drinking any warm fluids before breakfast."

3. What is the best diagnostic test to use when attempting to diagnose acute appendicitis?

    1. ultrasound

    2. x-ray

    3. intravenous pyelogram

    4. urinalysis

4. A urine output of less than _____ mL/hr indicates hypovolemia, decreased cardiac output, and impaired tissue perfusion.

    1. 30

    2. 50

    3. 60

    4. 75

5. Identify the diarrheal illness caused by ingesting raw or improperly cooked meat, eggs, and dairy products in which symptoms develop 8–48 hours after ingestion.

    1. shigellosis

    2. travelers' diarrhea

    3. cholera

    4. salmonellosis

6. Which statement indicates the need for further education about common bowel infections?

    1. "Giardiasis is a protozoal infection of the proximal small intestine."

    2. "Helminths are parasitic worms capable of causing bowel infections."

    3. "Amebiasis is an infection that attacks only the small bowel."

    4. "Coccidiosis secretes an enterotoxin that causes watery diarrhea."

7. Which action indicates that the patient is not correctly managing his inflammatory bowel disease (IBD)?

    1. The patient has added Ensure® to his diet.

    2. The patient reports drinking less than 1 quart of fluid per day.

    3. The patient takes medication as ordered by his physician.

    4. The patient has started smoking cessation classes.

8. How must patients with celiac disease adjust their diets?

    1. increase in lactose

    2. addition of fats

    3. decrease in calories

    4. elimination of gluten

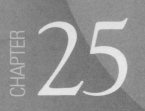

Nursing Care of Patients with **Gallbladder, Liver,** and **Pancreatic Disorders**

LEARNING OUTCOMES

1. Describe the pathophysiology of commonly occurring disorders of the gallbladder, liver, and exocrine pancreas.
2. Use knowledge of normal anatomy and physiology to understand the manifestations and effects of biliary, hepatic, and pancreatic disorders.
3. Relate changes in normal assessment data to the pathophysiology and manifestations of gallbladder, liver, and exocrine pancreatic disorders.

CLINICAL COMPETENCIES

1. Assess the health status of patients with gallbladder, liver, or pancreatic disease, eliciting patient values, preferences, and expressed needs when assessing, planning, and implementing care.
2. Monitor for, recognize, document, and report expected and unexpected manifestations in patients with gallbladder, liver, or pancreatic disease.
3. Integrate interprofessional measures into nursing care and teaching of the patient with a gallbladder, liver, or pancreatic disorder.
4. Provide safe, patient-centered nursing care for the patient who has surgery of the gallbladder, liver, or pancreas.
5. Integrate psychosocial, cultural, and spiritual considerations into the plan of care for a patient with a gallbladder, liver, or pancreatic disorder.
6. Use evidence-based practice, technology, and information management tools to develop, implement, evaluate, and, as needed, revise the plan of care for patients with disorders of the gallbladder, liver, or pancreas.
7. Provide appropriate evidence-based patient and family teaching to promote, maintain, and restore functional health status for patients with gallbladder, liver, and pancreatic disorders.

TERMS MATCHING

Place the letter of the correct definition in the space next to each term.

1. _____ ascites

2. _____ biliary colic

3. _____ cholecystitis

4. _____ cholelithiasis

5. _____ cirrhosis

6. _____ esophageal varices

7. _____ hepatitis

8. _____ jaundice

9. _____ pancreatitis

10. _____ paracentesis

11. _____ portal hypertension

12. _____ portal systemic encephalopathy

13. _____ steatorrhea

A. The formation of stones in the gallbladder or biliary duct system

B. Impaired consciousness and mental status due to the accumulation of toxic waste products in the blood as blood bypasses the congested liver

C. Elevated pressure in the portal venous system that causes rerouting of blood to adjoining lower pressure vessels

D. A procedure where fluid is aspirated from the peritoneal cavity

E. Enlarged thin-walled veins that form in the submucosa of the esophagus; formed when blood is shunted from the portal system due to portal hypertension

F. Excess accumulation of plasma-rich fluid in the abdominal cavity

G. Inflammation of the pancreas

H. Inflammation of the liver usually caused by a virus, although it may result from exposure to alcohol, drugs and toxins, or other pathogens

I. Yellow-to-orange color visible in the skin and mucous membranes

J. Inflammation of the gallbladder

K. Greasy, frothy, yellow stools resulting from excess fat in the feces

L. A severe, steady pain in the epigastric region or right upper quadrant of the abdomen

M. A progressive, irreversible disorder, eventually leading to liver failure; the end stage of chronic liver disease

FOCUSED STUDY

1. List 10 risk factors associated with the development of gallstones.

_____

_____

_____

_____

_____

2. Explain the physiological process of jaundice. List the three types of jaundice.

_____

_____

_____

_____

3. Describe the differences between the clinical manifestations associated with chronic versus acute pancreatitis.

_____

_____

_____

_____

_____

4. Describe two nursing interventions that can be performed for a patient who is experiencing acute pain related to cholelithiasis. Include a rationale for each intervention.

_____

_____

_____

_____

_____

CASE STUDY

Joseph Wales, a 62-year-old Black male, has been admitted with a diagnosis of acute pancreatitis. Six months ago he was diagnosed with cholelithiasis and had a laparoscopic cholecystectomy. Mr. Wales has a history of alcoholism. Answer the following questions based on your knowledge of caring for patients with acute pancreatitis.

1. What role does Mr. Wales's past medical history play in his current episode of acute pancreatitis?

2. What clinical manifestations are associated with acute pancreatitis?

3. The nurse is monitoring Mr. Wales for the development of complications related to acute pancreatitis. What are some complications of acute pancreatitis?

4. What are common nursing diagnoses associated with acute pancreatitis?

5. The nurse reviews Mr. Wales's laboratory results. Which laboratory results does the nurse expect to be abnormal?

6. Describe discharge teaching the nurse should provide for Mr. Wales.

CARE PLAN CRITICAL-THINKING ACTIVITY

Please refer to the case study and nursing care plan exercise: A Patient with Cholelithiasis included in your textbook to answer the following questions.

1. What role did Mrs. Red Wing's genetic makeup play in the development of cholelithiasis?

2. What nursing interventions may be used to deal with Mrs. Red Wing's recent weight loss?

SHORT ANSWERS

Fill in the blanks regarding the various types of viral hepatitis.

Virus	Hepatitis A (HAV)	Hepatitis B (HBV)	Hepatitis C (HCV)	Hepatitis D (HDV)	Hepatitis E (HEV)
Mode of transmission					
Incubation (in weeks)					
Onset					
Carrier state					
Possible complications					
Laboratory findings					

REVIEW QUESTIONS

1. The nurse knows that most gallstones consist primarily of which substance?
   1. cholesterol
   2. bile salts
   3. calcium
   4. lecithin

2. The nurse is assessing a patient with a diagnosis of acute cholecystitis. Which finding is the least likely clinical manifestation?
   1. nausea
   2. fever
   3. right upper quadrant pain
   4. diarrhea

3. The patient presents with abnormal liver function studies and impaired consciousness. What problem is the patient most likely experiencing?
   1. portal systemic encephalopathy
   2. ascites
   3. hepatorenal syndrome
   4. splenomegaly

4. Administering the hepatitis B vaccine protects the patient against what other form of the disease?
   1. hepatitis A
   2. hepatitis C
   3. hepatitis delta
   4. hepatitis E

5. The nurse is creating a care plan for the patient with liver trauma. Which nursing diagnosis would be unexpected in the care of this patient?
   1. *Deficient Fluid Volume Related to Hemorrhage*
   2. *Risk for Infection Related to Wound or Abdominal Contamination*
   3. *Risk for Bleeding Related to Impaired Coagulation*
   4. *Altered Body Image Related to Bruising*

6. The patient has developed pancreatic cancer. Which factor is not a known risk for the development of pancreatic cancer?
   1. occupational exposure to industrial chemicals
   2. a low-fat diet
   3. diagnosis of diabetes mellitus 7 years ago
   4. history of smoking two packs per day for the last 19 years

26 Assessing the **Renal System**

LEARNING OUTCOMES

1. Describe the anatomy, physiology, and functions of the renal system.
2. Identify specific topics for consideration during a health history interview of the patient with health problems involving the renal system.
3. Describe techniques used to assess the integrity and function of the renal system.
4. Give examples of genetic disorders of the renal system.
5. Describe normal variations in assessment findings for the older adult.
6. Identify abnormal findings that may indicate alterations in urinary elimination.

CLINICAL COMPETENCIES

1. Conduct and document a health history for patients who have or are at risk for alterations in renal function, eliciting patient values, preferences, and expressed needs as part of the interview.
2. Conduct and document a physical assessment of the renal system, demonstrating sensitivity and respect for the diversity of human experience.
3. Monitor the results of diagnostic tests and communicate abnormal findings within the interprofessional team.

TERMS MATCHING

Place the letter of the correct definition in the space next to each item.

1. _____ dysuria

2. _____ hematuria

3. _____ micturition

4. _____ nocturia

5. _____ urea

A. Voiding two or more times at night

B. An end product of protein metabolism, eliminated in the urine

C. Pain experienced with urination

D. The process of urinating or voiding

E. The presence of blood in the urine

FOCUSED STUDY

1. Discuss the organs of the urinary system.

_____

_____

_____

2. Summarize diagnostic tests for the urinary system.

_____

_____

_____

3. Explain the formation of urine.

_____

_____

_____

CASE STUDY

Anne Sutter is a 64-year-old female patient admitted to the nursing unit. Her skin and mucous membranes are pale. She also has tenderness and pain on percussion of the costovertebral angle.

1. Explain the functions of the kidney.

2. What could tenderness and pain on percussion of the costovertebral angle suggest?

3. What could pallor of the skin and mucous membranes indicate?

CROSSWORD PUZZLE

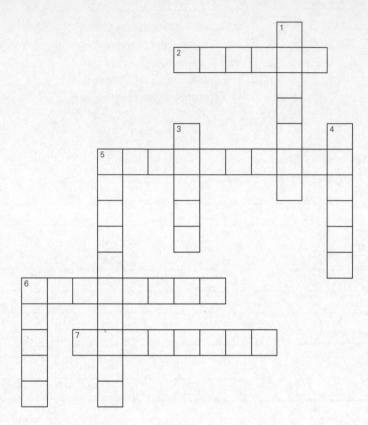

Across

2   Channels urine from the kidney to the bladder
5   The test used to directly visualize the bladder wall
6   Urine remaining in the bladder after voiding
7   The substance necessary for the absorption of calcium

Down

1   The functional unit of the kidney
3   The color of normal urine
4   Milky urine is the result of this
5   The by-product of muscle breakdown that is excreted by the kidney
6   Acts on a plasma globulin, angiotensinogen, to release angiotensin I, which in turn is converted to angiotensin II

REVIEW QUESTIONS

1. The patient contacts the ambulatory care clinic with concerns about her urine appearing discolored. The nursing interview determines that the urine is a bright orange color. Which question by the nurse is indicated at this time?
   1. "Are you currently sexually active?"
   2. "Is your dietary intake high in saturated fats?"
   3. "Are you taking iron supplements?"
   4. "Are you currently taking any medications?"

2. Which process is a function of the kidney?
   1. to form urine
   2. to conserve metabolic waste products
   3. to destroy nutrients
   4. to secrete solutes

3. Which statement about glomerular filtration is true?
   1. Hydrostatic pressure forces fluid and solutes through a membrane.
   2. It is a passive, selective process.
   3. Glomerular filtration rate (GFR) is not influenced by the total surface area available for filtration.
   4. The glomerulus is less efficient than most capillary beds.

4. Urine is composed, by volume, of about _____% water and _____% solutes.
   1. 95; 5
   2. 85; 15
   3. 75; 25
   4. 65; 35

5. Which statement is correct about renal proteins?
   1. The stimulus for the production of erythropoietin by the kidneys is increased oxygen delivery to kidney cells.
   2. Erythropoietin stimulates the bone marrow to produce red blood cells in response to tissue hypoxia.
   3. Hormones activated or synthesized by the kidneys include the active form of vitamin E, erythropoietin, and natriuretic hormone.
   4. Vitamin D is necessary for the absorption of calcium and phosphate by the large intestine.

6. What are the layers of the bladder wall (from internal to external)?
   1. the epithelial mucosa lining the inside, the connective tissue submucosa, the smooth muscle layer, and the fibrous outer layer
   2. the fibrous outer layer, the connective tissue submucosa, the epithelial mucosa lining the inside, and the smooth muscle layer
   3. the fibrous outer layer, the epithelial mucosa lining the inside, the connective tissue submucosa, and the smooth muscle layer
   4. the connective tissue submucosa, the epithelial mucosa lining the inside, the smooth muscle layer, and the fibrous outer layer

7. Which statement about the bladder is correct?
   1. "It holds about 600–800 mL of urine before internal pressure rises and signals the need to empty the bladder through micturition."
   2. "It is posterior to the symphysis pubis and serves as a storage site for urine."
   3. "In females, the bladder lies immediately in front of the rectum."
   4. "Openings for the ureters and the urethra are outside the bladder."

8. The nurse is reviewing the patient's history and physical information and notes the physician's indication that the patient has been experiencing hematuria. What does the nurse recognize about the patient?
   1. There is blood in the patient's urine.
   2. The patient gets up frequently at night to urinate.
   3. The patient is voiding excessive amounts of urine.
   4. Voiding is painful.

9. The nurse is reviewing the patient's most recent urinalysis. Which finding indicates the need for further action?
   1. light straw color
   2. pH of 5.5
   3. WBCs 3
   4. ketones +1

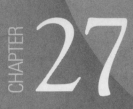

27 Nursing Care of Patients with **Urinary Tract Disorders**

LEARNING OUTCOMES

1. Identify populations at risk for common urinary tract disorders and behaviors that increase the risk.
2. Explain the pathophysiology of common urinary tract disorders.
3. Describe the manifestations of urinary tract disorders, relating manifestations to the pathophysiology of the disorder.
4. Discuss the nursing implications of medications and treatments prescribed for patients with urinary tract disorders.
5. Describe invasive and surgical procedures used in treating urinary tract disorders.

CLINICAL COMPETENCIES

1. Assess the functional health status of patients with urinary tract disorders, using data and expressed needs, values, and preferences to determine priority nursing diagnoses and select individualized nursing interventions.
2. Identify, document, and monitor abnormal or unexpected changes in patient status, communicating information within the interprofessional team as appropriate.
3. Use evidence-based research to plan and implement nursing care for patients with urinary tract disorders.
4. Integrate the interprofessional plan of care into care for patients with urinary tract disorders.
5. Knowledgeably and safely administer prescribed medications and treatments for patients with urinary tract disorders.
6. Provide safe and effective nursing care for patients undergoing invasive procedures or surgery of the urinary tract.
7. Plan and provide appropriate teaching for prevention and self-care of urinary tract disorders.
8. Use evidence-based guidelines to reduce the incidence of healthcare-associated urinary tract infections.
9. Participate in studies and projects to improve the quality and safety of care for patients with urinary tract disorders.
10. Document care in the electronic medical record and use information management tools to monitor outcomes of care.

TERMS MATCHING

Place the letter of the correct definition in the space next to each item.

1. _____ cystectomy

2. _____ cystitis

3. _____ dysuria

4. _____ hematuria

5. _____ hydronephrosis

6. _____ lithiasis

7. _____ lithotripsy

8. _____ neurogenic bladder

9. _____ nocturia

10. _____ pyelonephritis

11. _____ renal colic

12. _____ ureteral stent

13. _____ ureteroplasty

14. _____ urgency

15. _____ urinary calculi

16. _____ urinary diversion

17. _____ urinary incontinence (UI)

A. Distention of the renal pelvis and calyces

B. Crushing of renal calculi

C. Stones in the urinary tract

D. Upper urinary tract inflammation affecting the kidney and renal pelvis

E. Dysfunctional urinary bladder due to lesion of central or peripheral nervous system

F. Surgical removal of the bladder

G. A thin catheter inserted into the ureter to provide for urine flow

H. A sudden, compelling need to urinate

I. The involuntary loss of urine

J. Acute, severe flank pain that develops when a stone obstructs the ureter, causing ureteral spasm

K. Inflammation of the urinary bladder

L. Stone formation

M. Surgical repair of a ureter

N. Blood in urine

O. Voiding two or more times at night

P. Painful or difficult urination

Q. The surgical technique used to reroute the normal flow of urine and provide for urine collection and drainage

FOCUSED STUDY

1. Summarize the surgical procedures used to treat urinary tract disorders.

_____

_____

_____

_____

2. Discuss three diagnostic tests used to diagnose disorders that affect the urinary tract.

_____

_____

3. Summarize the pathophysiology of common urinary tract disorders.

_____

_____

4. List the risk factors for urinary tract infection (UTI).

_____

_____

_____

CASE STUDY

Christine Scott is a 37-year-old female patient who came to the clinic today. She is complaining of dysuria, hematuria, and urgency. She is diagnosed with cystitis. Answer the following questions based on your knowledge of cystitis.

1. Explain cystitis.

2. What can occur if cystitis is left untreated?

3. Why does cystitis occur more frequently in adult females?

4. List the manifestations of cystitis.

SHORT ANSWERS

Fill in the table regarding manifestations of acute pyelonephritis. Give examples of each.

Urinary	Systemic

REVIEW QUESTIONS

1. Which statement about urinary tract infections (UTIs) is correct?
   1. More than 10 million people are treated annually for UTI.
   2. Community-acquired UTIs are not common in young women and are unusual in men over the age of 50.
   3. Most community-acquired UTIs are caused by *Escherichia coli*, a common gram-positive enteral bacteria.
   4. Catheter-associated UTIs often involve other gram-negative bacteria such as *Proteus*, *Klebsiella*, *Serratia*, and *Pseudomonas*.

2. Which statement by a student nurse reflects the need for further clarification concerning the urinary tract?
   1. "The urinary tract is normally sterile below the urethra."
   2. "Adequate urine volume, a free flow from the kidneys through the urinary meatus, and complete bladder emptying are the most important mechanisms for maintaining sterility."
   3. "Pathogens that enter and contaminate the distal urethra are washed out during voiding."
   4. "Other defenses for maintaining sterile urine include its normal acidity and the bacteriostatic properties of the bladder and urethral cells."

3. Which type of incontinence is the loss of urine associated with increased intra-abdominal pressure during sneezing, coughing, or lifting in which the quantity of urine lost is usually small?
   1. urge
   2. stress
   3. overflow
   4. functional

4. Which statement would the nurse include when providing education to a patient who is receiving a urinary anti-infective?
   1. "These drugs are used along with hygiene practices to prevent recurrent urinary tract infection. Take as directed, even when no symptoms are present."
   2. "Drink 10–12 glasses of water or fluid per day while taking these drugs."
   3. "Take the drug before meals or food to reduce gastric effects and drink one glass of milk after taking the drug."
   4. "Nitrofurantoin (Furadantin®, Nitrofan) turns the urine blue. This is not harmful and subsides when the drug is discontinued."

5. When discussing the management of urolithiasis, the nurse should recommend which action?
   1. Collect and strain all urine, saving any stones.
   2. Do not report stone passage to the physician or bring the stone in for analysis.
   3. Report to physician only the changes in the amount of urine output.
   4. Increase fluid intake to 1,550–2,450 mL per day.

6. The nurse is evaluating a student nurse's understanding of bladder cancer. Which statement indicates a need for further teaching?
   1. An estimated 73,980 new cases of bladder cancer were diagnosed in the United States in 2012, and 14,880 people died as a result of the disease.
   2. The incidence of bladder cancer is about four times higher in women than it is in men and about twice as high in Whites as it is in Blacks.
   3. Cigarette smoking is the primary risk factor for bladder cancer.
   4. Most people who develop bladder cancer are over age 60.

7. Diet modifications are often prescribed to change the character of the urine and prevent further lithiasis. The nurse would explain that foods high in oxalate include
   1. beans and lentils, dried fruits, canned or smoked fish except tuna, flour, milk, and milk products.
   2. asparagus, beer and colas, beets, cabbage, celery, fruits, green beans, nuts, tea, and tomatoes.
   3. goose, organ meats, sardines and herring, venison; moderate consumption of beef, chicken, crab, pork, salmon, and veal.
   4. cheese, cranberries, eggs, grapes, meat and poultry, plums and prunes, tomatoes, and whole grains.

8. Which action is inappropriate for the nurse who is providing urinary stoma care?
   1. Remove old pouch, pulling it away from the skin gently. Use warm water or adhesive solvent to loosen the seal if necessary.
   2. Gather all supplies: a clean, disposable pouch; a liquid skin barrier or barrier ring; 4×4 gauze squares; a stoma guide; an adhesive solvent; clean gloves; and a clean washcloth.
   3. Cleanse skin around the stoma with soap and water, rinse, and pat or air-dry.
   4. Apply the bag with an opening no more than 3–4 mm wider than the outside of the stoma.

9. The nurse is discussing the following points with a patient to help prevent UTI and UI in an older adult. Which statement is correct?
   1. "Maintain a generous fluid intake. Increase fluid intake after the evening meal to reduce nocturia."
   2. "Perform pelvic muscle exercises (Kegel exercises) two times a day to increase perineal muscle tone."
   3. "Increase the consumption of caffeine-containing beverages (coffee, tea, colas), citrus juices, and artificially sweetened beverages that contain NutraSweet®."
   4. "Use behavioral techniques such as scheduled toileting, habit training, and bladder training to reduce the frequency of incontinence."

CHAPTER 28

Nursing Care of Patients with **Kidney Disorders**

LEARNING OUTCOMES

1. Describe the pathophysiology of common kidney disorders, relating pathophysiology to normal functions and manifestations of the disorder.
2. Discuss risk factors for kidney disorders and nursing measures to reduce these risks.
3. Explain diagnostic studies used to identify disorders of the kidneys and their effects.
4. Discuss the effects of and nursing implications for medications and treatments used for patients with kidney disorders.
5. Compare and contrast renal replacement therapies, including dialysis and kidney transplant, to manage acute kidney injury and chronic kidney disease.

CLINICAL COMPETENCIES

1. Assess and monitor the health status of patients with kidney disorders, recognizing and reporting unexpected manifestations or status changes.
2. Provide safe and effective nursing care for patients undergoing renal replacement therapies, surgery involving the kidneys, or renal transplant, respecting the patient's expressed needs, values, and preferences.
3. Using assessed data and current standards of practice, plan and implement evidence-based nursing care for patients with renal disorders using research and best practices.
4. Collaborate and coordinate with the patient and other members of the interprofessional team to prioritize and implement care.
5. Provide teaching appropriate to the individual and situation for patients with kidney disorders.
6. Evaluate patient responses to care, revising the plan of care as needed to promote, maintain, or restore functional health status for patients with renal disorders.
7. Participate in studies and projects to improve outcomes for patients with acute or chronic kidney disorders.
8. Apply technology and information management tools to support safe processes of care for patients with kidney disorders.

TERMS MATCHING

Place the letter of the correct definition in the space next to each item.

1. _____ acute kidney injury (AKI)

2. _____ acute tubular necrosis (ATN)

3. _____ azotemia

4. _____ chronic kidney disease (CKD)

5. _____ dialysis

6. _____ glomerular filtration rate (GFR)

7. _____ glomerulonephritis

8. _____ hematuria

9. _____ hemodialysis

10. _____ kidney failure

11. _____ nephrectomy

12. _____ nephrotic syndrome

13. _____ oliguria

14. _____ peritoneal dialysis

15. _____ proteinuria

16. _____ ultrafiltration

17. _____ uremia

A. The rate at which plasma is filtered through the glomeruli of the kidney

B. The diffusion of solute molecules across a semipermeable membrane

C. Abnormal proteins in the urine

D. Blood in the urine

E. Removal of the kidney

F. Urine output of less than 400 mL in 24 hours

G. A rapid decline in renal function

H. A condition in which the kidneys are unable to remove accumulated metabolites from the blood

I. The presence of kidney damage for 3 or more months

J. Uses the peritoneum surrounding the abdominal cavity as the dialyzing membrane

K. A condition marked by massive proteinuria, hypoalbuminemia, hyperlipidemia, and edema

L. Removal of excess body water using a hydrostatic pressure gradient

M. A syndrome of abrupt and progressive decline in tubular and glomerular function

N. A procedure in which blood passes through a semipermeable membrane filter outside the body

O. Inflammation of the glomerular capillary membrane

P. A term meaning "urine in the blood" that refers to the syndrome or group of symptoms associated with end-stage renal disease (ESRD)

Q. Increased blood levels of nitrogenous waste

FOCUSED STUDY

1. Summarize the dialysis procedures used to manage acute and chronic renal failure.

_____

_____

_____

_____

2. Define polycystic kidney disease.

_____

_____

3. List the diagnostic studies used when polycystic kidney disease is suspected.

_____

_____

_____

_____

_____

4. List the risk factors for acute renal artery thrombosis.

_____

_____

_____

_____

_____

CASE STUDY

Brent Brelle is a 67-year-old male patient admitted to the unit this morning. The physician thinks he might have a renal tumor. His spouse Nancy has several questions about his condition for the nurse. Answer the following questions based on your knowledge of renal tumors.

1. "Why didn't my husband have any signs or symptoms until the last few days?"

2. "What tests might the physician order to determine whether Brent has a renal tumor?"

3. "What is the treatment of choice for a renal tumor?"

SHORT ANSWERS

List possible manifestations associated with each of the following electrolyte imbalances.

Electrolyte Imbalance	Manifestations
Hyperkalemia	
Hyponatremia	
Hyperphosphatemia	

REVIEW QUESTIONS

1. Which statement about glomerular disorders is false?
   1. "Glomerular disorders and diseases are the leading cause of chronic kidney disease in the United States."
   2. "Hematuria, proteinuria, and hypertension often are early manifestations of glomerular disorders."
   3. "Acute poststreptococcal glomerulonephritis (also called acute proliferative glomerulonephritis) is the least common primary glomerular disorder."
   4. "Diabetes mellitus, hypertension, and systemic lupus erythematosus (SLE) are common causes of primary glomerulonephritis."

2. Which statement regarding polycystic kidney disease indicates a need for further teaching?
   1. "This is a slowly progressive disease."
   2. "Symptoms usually develop by age 40 to 50."
   3. "Common manifestations include flank pain, microscopic or gross hematuria, proteinuria, polyuria, and nocturia."
   4. "The progression to end-stage renal disease tends to occur more rapidly in women than in men."

3. When discussing the nutrition and fluid management with a male patient of average size who has chronic kidney disease, the nurse would recommend which strategy?
   1. Increase water intake to make urine more dilute.
   2. Limit sodium to 4 grams a day.
   3. Increase potassium intake to more than 80 mEq/day.
   4. Limit daily protein intake to approximately 40 grams a day.

4. A nurse is planning a seminar about dialysis. Which statement should not be included in this seminar?
   1. "For the patient who is not a candidate for renal transplantation or who has had a transplant failure, dialysis is life-sustaining."
   2. "Hemodialysis for end-stage renal disease (ESRD) typically is done three times a week for a total of 9–12 hours."
   3. "Patients on long-term dialysis have a higher risk for complications and death than does the general population."
   4. "Serum triglyceride levels decrease with peritoneal dialysis."

5. Which situation is least likely to result in acute kidney injury (AKI)?
   1. major trauma or surgery
   2. infection
   3. hemorrhage
   4. emotional stress

6. A nurse is evaluating a patient's understanding of chronic kidney disease (CKD). Which statement indicates a need for further teaching?
   1. "The incidence of CKD and ESRD is significantly higher in people aged 65 and older."
   2. "People of Hispanic origin have a higher incidence of CKD and ESRD than do non-Hispanics."
   3. "Hypertension is the leading cause of CKD, followed by diabetes mellitus."
   4. "Men are more likely to be affected by CKD and ESRD than are women."

7. The nurse who is evaluating a kidney transplant class recognizes that further teaching is necessary when a participant makes which statement?
   1. "The donor kidney is placed in the upper abdominal cavity of the recipient, and the renal artery, vein, and ureter are anastomosed."
   2. "Kidney transplant improves both survival rate and quality of life for the patient with end-stage renal disease (ESRD)."
   3. "Most transplanted kidneys are obtained from deceased donors."
   4. "Hypertension is a possible complication of a kidney transplant."

8. Which phase is not typically included in the course of acute renal failure due to acute tubular necrosis (ATN)?
   1. intrarenal
   2. initiation
   3. maintenance
   4. recovery

29

Assessing the Cardiovascular and Lymphatic Systems

LEARNING OUTCOMES

1. Describe the anatomy, physiology, and functions of the cardiovascular and lymphatic systems.
2. Describe normal variations in cardiovascular assessment findings for the older adult.
3. Give examples of genetic disorders of the cardiovascular system.
4. Identify specific topics for consideration during a health history assessment interview of the patient with cardiovascular or lymphatic disorders.
5. Explain techniques used to assess cardiovascular and lymphatic structure and function.
6. Identify manifestations of impaired cardiovascular structure and functions.

CLINICAL COMPETENCIES

1. Complete a health history for patients having alterations in the structure and functions of the cardiovascular or lymphatic systems.
2. Conduct and document a physical assessment of cardiovascular and lymphatic status.
3. Assess an ECG strip and identify normal rhythm and cardiac events and abnormal cardiac rhythm.
4. Monitor the results of diagnostic tests and communicate abnormal findings within the interprofessional team.

TERMS MATCHING

Place the letter of the correct definition in the space next to each term.

1. _____ apical impulse

2. _____ cardiac index (CI)

3. _____ cardiac output (CO)

4. _____ dysrhythmia

5. _____ heave

6. _____ hemostasis

7. _____ ischemic

8. _____ Korotkoff's sounds

9. _____ lift

10. _____ lymphadenopathy

11. _____ lymphedema

12. _____ orthostatic hypotension

13. _____ retraction

14. _____ thrill

15. _____ thrust

A. An abnormal heart rate or rhythm

B. Control of bleeding

C. A decrease in systolic blood pressure (BP) of more than 10–15 mmHg and a drop in diastolic BP upon standing

D. The cardiac output that is adjusted for the patient's body size; provides meaningful data about the heart's ability to perfuse the tissues; a more accurate indicator of the effectiveness of the circulation

E. A visible pulsation

F. The amount of blood pumped by the ventricles into the pulmonary and systemic circulations in 1 minute

G. A palpable vibration over the precordium or an artery

H. Enlargement of lymph nodes

I. The sounds that can be auscultated when the nurse takes the patient's blood pressure

J. Deprived of oxygen

K. An excessive thrust; also known as lifts

L. Edema of an extremity due to accumulated lymph

M. A pulling in of tissue

N. A normal, visible pulsation in the area of the midclavicular line in the left fifth intercostal space

O. A more sustained thrust than normal; also known as heaves

FOCUSED STUDY

1. Describe the cardiac cycle.

_____

_____

_____

2. Describe how the following factors can influence arterial blood pressure.

Sympathetic and parasympathetic nervous systems: _____

_____

Baroreceptors and chemoreceptors: _____

_____

Kidneys: _____

_____

Temperature: _____

_____

Chemicals, hormones, and drugs: _____

_____

Diet: _____

_____

3. Explain how red blood cells are destroyed.

_____

_____

_____

4. List four topics the nurse should discuss with the patient regarding possible genetic influences on the patient's health.

_____

_____

_____

_____

CASE STUDY

Jonathan Drake is a 63-year-old male patient who is scheduled for an electrocardiogram and a treadmill test (stress test). Mr. Drake has had recent episodes of chest pain with activity. Answer the following questions based on your knowledge of caring for patients who require a cardiovascular assessment and diagnostic testing.

1. What is an electrocardiogram (ECG)?

2. How are ECG waveforms recorded?

3. The experienced nurse who works in cardiovascular testing has been asked to interpret Mr. Drake's ECG results. What six steps are used to interpret an ECG?

4. Mr. Drake is preparing for the stress test. About what should the nurse educate Mr. Drake prior to the test?

5. During the stress test, Mr. Drake complains of chest pain. What are some common ways that patients describe chest pain?

6. With further testing, the physician determines that Mr. Drake's heart rate is 92 beats per minute and his stroke volume is 40 mL/beat. Calculate Mr. Drake's cardiac output.

7. Mr. Drake has blood drawn to determine his lipid levels. His cholesterol is 392 mg/dL, and triglycerides are 210 mg/dL. What are normal values?

SHORT ANSWERS

Fill in the blanks, noting the significance of each age-related change in the patient.

Age-Related Change	Significance
Myocardium: ↓ efficiency and contractibility Sinus node: ↑ in thickness of shell surrounding the node and ↓ in the number of pacemaker cells	
Left ventricle: slight hypertrophy, prolonged isometric contraction phase and relaxation time; ↑ time for diastolic filling and systolic emptying cycle	
Valves and blood vessels: elongated and dilated aorta, thicker and more rigid valves, and increase in resistance to peripheral blood flow by 1% per year	
Bone marrow: ↓ ability of bone marrow to respond to need for increased RBCs, WBCs, and platelets	
Blood vessels: Tunica intima: fibrosis, calcium and lipid accumulation, cellular proliferation Tunica media: thins, elastin fibers calcify; increase in calcium results in stiffening; baroreceptor function is impaired, and peripheral resistance increases	
Immune system: impaired function of B and T lymphocytes; ↓ production of antibodies	

REVIEW QUESTIONS

1. What covers the entire heart and great vessels and then folds over to form the parietal layer that lines the pericardium and adheres to the heart surface?
   1. endocardium
   2. myocardium
   3. epicardium
   4. parietal pericardium

2. Which statement made by the student nurse indicates the need for further education?
   1. "The right atrium receives deoxygenated blood from the veins of the body."
   2. "The left ventricle receives deoxygenated blood from the left atrium and pumps it through the pulmonary artery to the pulmonary capillary bed for oxygenation."
   3. "The left atrium receives freshly oxygenated blood from the lungs through the pulmonary veins."
   4. "The superior vena cava returns blood from the body area above the diaphragm, the inferior vena cava returns blood from the body below the diaphragm, and the coronary sinus drains blood from the heart."

3. The greater the volume, the greater the stretch of the cardiac muscle fibers and the greater the force with which the fibers contract to accomplish emptying. This principle is called _____ law of the heart.
   1. Stuart's
   2. Starling's
   3. Sarton's
   4. Schell's

4. Which statement by a student nurse reflects an accurate understanding regarding the conduction system of the heart?
   1. The AV node acts as the normal "pacemaker" of the heart, usually generating an impulse 60–100 times per minute.
   2. The AV node is located at the junction of the superior vena cava and right atrium.
   3. The cellular action potential serves as the basis for electrocardiography, a diagnostic test of cardiac function.
   4. The electrical stimulus decreases the permeability of the cell membrane, which creates an action potential (electrical potential).

5. Which condition may lead to an increase in red blood cell production? **Select all that apply.**
   1. coronary artery disease
   2. renal failure
   3. emphysema
   4. cirrhosis
   5. pneumonia

6. Which statement indicates the need for further education regarding white blood cells?
   1. Neutrophils are active phagocytes.
   2. Immature neutrophils are called bands.
   3. Lymphocytes are phagocytic cells that mature into macrophages.
   4. Basophils and eosinophils increase in number during allergic reactions.

CHAPTER 30

Nursing Care of Patients with **Coronary Heart Disease**

LEARNING OUTCOMES

1. Discuss the coronary circulation and electrical properties of the heart.
2. Compare and contrast the pathophysiology and manifestations of coronary heart disease and common cardiac dysrhythmias.
3. Describe interprofessional and nursing care for patients with coronary heart disease and/or cardiac dysrhythmias.
4. Relate the outcomes of diagnostic tests and procedures to the pathophysiology of cardiac disorders and implications for patient responses to the disorder.
5. Discuss nursing implications for medications and treatments used to prevent and treat coronary heart disease and dysrhythmias.
6. Describe nursing care for the patient undergoing diagnostic testing, an interventional procedure, or surgery for coronary heart disease or a dysrhythmia.

CLINICAL COMPETENCIES

1. Assess the functional health status of patients with coronary heart disease and/or a dysrhythmia, including the impact of the disorder on the patient's ability to perform activities of daily living and usual tasks.
2. Use knowledge of the normal anatomy and physiology of the heart in caring for patients with coronary heart disease.
3. Monitor patients with coronary heart disease or dysrhythmias for expected and unexpected manifestations, reporting and recording findings as indicated.
4. Use assessed data to select nursing diagnoses, determine priorities of care, and develop and implement individualized nursing interventions for patients with coronary heart disease and dysrhythmias.
5. Administer medications and treatments for patients with coronary heart disease and dysrhythmias safely and knowledgably.
6. Integrate interprofessional care into nursing care planning and implementation for patients with coronary heart disease and dysrhythmias.
7. Provide appropriate teaching for prevention, health promotion, and self-care related to coronary heart disease and dysrhythmias.
8. Evaluate the effectiveness of nursing interventions, revising or modifying the plan of care as needed to promote, maintain, or restore functional health for patients with coronary heart disease or dysrhythmias.

TERMS MATCHING

Place the letter of the correct definition in the space next to each term.

1. _____ acute coronary syndrome (ACS)
2. _____ acute myocardial infarction (AMI)
3. _____ angina pectoris
4. _____ atherosclerosis
5. _____ atrial kick
6. _____ cardiac arrest
7. _____ cardiac rehabilitation
8. _____ cardiovascular disease (CVD)
9. _____ collateral channels
10. _____ coronary heart disease (CHD)
11. _____ dysrhythmia
12. _____ ectopic beats
13. _____ heart block
14. _____ ischemia
15. _____ pacemaker
16. _____ paroxysmal
17. _____ sudden cardiac death (SCD)

A. Connections between small arteries

B. Chest pain that results from reduced coronary blood flow, which causes a temporary imbalance between myocardial blood supply and demand

C. Heart disease caused by impaired blood flow to the myocardium

D. Myocardial tissue death

E. A block in the heart's normal conduction pathways

F. Deficient blood flow to tissue resulting in reduced oxygen delivery

G. A form of arteriosclerosis in which deposits of fat and fibrin obstruct and harden the arteries

H. Abnormal heart rate or rhythm

I. Sudden failure of the heart to pump

J. Abrupt onset and termination

K. A long-term program that includes medical evaluation, education, exercise, counseling, and risk factor modification; designed to reduce the psychologic and physical effects associated with cardiac illness

L. An unexpected death that occurs within 1 hour of the onset of cardiovascular symptoms

M. Delivery of an additional bolus of blood to the ventricles resulting from atrial systole; occurs just prior to ventricular systole

N. Impulses originating outside normal conduction pathways of the heart; this interrupts the normal conduction sequence and may not initiate a normal muscle contraction

O. A pulse generator used to provide an electrical stimulus to the heart when the heart fails to generate or conduct its own at a rate that maintains the cardiac output

P. A generic term for disorders of the heart and blood vessels

Q. A condition of unstable and severe cardiac ischemia

FOCUSED STUDY

1. Describe coronary circulation.

   _____

   _____

   _____

2. Briefly describe the following diagnostic tests that can be performed to diagnose or assess risk factors associated with coronary heart disease.

   Total serum cholesterol: _____

   _____

   C-reactive protein: _____

   _____

   Ankle-brachial blood pressure index: _____

   _____

   Exercise electrocardiogram (ECG) testing: _____

   _____

Electron beam computed tomography (EBCT): _____

_____

Myocardial perfusion imaging: _____

_____

3. List the medications that can be used to treat acute and chronic types of angina. Briefly describe how each type of medication works.

_____

_____

_____

_____

_____

_____

_____

4. Discuss the nursing interventions that should be included in the care plan of a patient who is experiencing acute chest pain. Include the rationale for each intervention.

_____

_____

_____

_____

_____

_____

CASE STUDY

Bradley Baldwin's elderly mother was recently diagnosed with coronary heart disease. He and his mother have created a list of questions to ask during a scheduled office visit. Answer the following questions based on your understanding of coronary heart disease.

1. What are some modifiable and nonmodifiable risk factors for coronary heart disease (CHD)?

2. What are atheromas?

3. What are some characteristics of metabolic syndrome?

4. Mr. Baldwin received training on how to perform cardiopulmonary resuscitation (CPR) 10 months ago. He asks the nurse to refresh his memory about how to perform CPR.

5. Mr. Baldwin's mother states, "I quit smoking 3 months ago. Will that have any effect on my lipid levels?" How should the nurse respond?

6. Mr. Baldwin requests information about how eating fish can reduce his mother's risk factors.

7. Mr. Baldwin's mother requests information about how exercise can reduce her risk factors.

CARE PLAN CRITICAL-THINKING ACTIVITY

Refer to the case study and nursing care plan for Elisa Vasquez in your textbook.

1. Explain synchronized cardioversion.

_____

_____

_____

2. What could occur if Ms. Vasquez's heart continues to beat at the current rate?

_____

_____

_____

3. Why is it important to know that Ms. Vasquez had rheumatic fever as a child?

_____

_____

SHORT ANSWERS

Fill in the blanks regarding dietary recommendations to reduce CHD risk.

Nutrient	Recommendation
Calories	
Total fat	
Saturated fats	
Polyunsaturated fats	
Monounsaturated fats	
Cholesterol	
Carbohydrate (primarily complex carbohydrates such as whole grains, fruits, and vegetables)	
Dietary fiber	
Protein	

REVIEW QUESTIONS

1. The nurse is teaching a course about coronary heart disease (CHD). The nurse recognizes that further teaching is necessary when which statement is made by a participant in the class?
  1. "CHD is caused by impaired blood flow to the myocardium."
  2. "CHD is always associated with signs or symptoms."
  3. "CHD affects 16.3 million people in the United States and causes more than 405,000 deaths annually."
  4. "Accumulation of atherosclerotic plaque in the coronary arteries is the usual cause of CHD."

2. The patient has been diagnosed with metabolic syndrome. Which is an unexpected finding during the nurse's assessment of this patient?
  1. hypertension
  2. elevated fasting blood glucose
  3. high HDL
  4. abdominal obesity

3. A nurse is providing education to a patient about antianginal medications. Which statement would demonstrate to the nurse that the patient needs further education?

    1. "If the first nitrate dose does not relieve angina within 5 minutes, I'll take a second dose. After 5 more minutes, I may take a third dose if needed. If the pain is unrelieved or lasts 20 minutes or longer, I'll seek medical assistance immediately."

    2. "I'll carry a supply of nitroglycerin tablets with me. I should dissolve sublingual nitroglycerin tablets under my tongue or between the upper lip and gum. I cannot eat, drink, or smoke until the tablet is completely dissolved."

    3. "I'll keep the sublingual tablets in a small envelope that will fit in my wallet and I'll replace the supply every 12 months."

    4. "I'll rotate the ointment or transdermal patch application sites. I'll apply to a hairless area; I'll spread ointment evenly without rubbing or massaging. I'll remove the patch or residual ointment at bedtime daily and apply a fresh dose in the morning."

4. Which situation is a cause of sudden cardiac death? **Select all that apply.**

    1. dissecting aortic aneurysm

    2. choking

    3. mitral valve prolapse

    4. pulmonary embolism

    5. myocarditis

5. When a nurse is performing CPR on an adult patient, which action is correct?

    1. Open the airway using the head-thrust, chin-thrust maneuver.

    2. Check the brachial artery for a pulse.

    3. Provide two breaths after every 30 compressions.

    4. Assess for responsiveness by flicking the patient's foot.

6. What is a deficient blood flow to tissue that may be caused by partial obstruction of a coronary artery, a coronary artery spasm, or a thrombus?

    1. atrial kick

    2. angina pectoris

    3. ectopic beats

    4. ischemia

7. A nurse is presenting a seminar about myocardial infarction (MI) to patients who have been diagnosed with coronary heart disease. Which statement by a patient demonstrates the need for further teaching?

    1. "MI occurs when blood flow to a portion of cardiac muscle is completely blocked, which results in prolonged tissue ischemia and irreversible cell damage."

    2. "MI usually affects the right ventricle because it is the major "workhorse" of the heart; its muscle mass and oxygen demands are greater."

    3. "MIs are described by the damaged area of the heart."

    4. "Risk factors for MI are the same as those for coronary heart disease: age, gender, heredity, race, smoking, obesity, hyperlipidemia, hypertension, diabetes, sedentary lifestyle, and diet, among others."

Nursing Care of Patients with Cardiac Disorders

LEARNING OUTCOMES

1. Compare and contrast the etiology, pathophysiology, and manifestations of common cardiac disorders, including heart failure, structural disorders, and inflammatory disorders.
2. Explain risk factors and preventive measures for cardiac disorders such as heart failure, inflammatory disorders, and valve disorders.
3. Discuss indications for and management of patients with hemodynamic monitoring.
4. Discuss the effects and nursing implications for medications commonly prescribed for patients with cardiac disorders.
5. Describe nursing care for the patient undergoing cardiac surgery or cardiac transplant.

CLINICAL COMPETENCIES

1. Apply knowledge of normal cardiac anatomy and physiology and assessment techniques in caring for patients with cardiac disorders.
2. Assess the functional health status of patients with cardiac disorders, documenting and reporting deviations from expected findings.
3. Based on patient assessment and knowledge of the disorder, determine priority nursing diagnoses.
4. Plan, prioritize, and provide evidence-based, individualized care for patients with cardiac disorders.
5. Safely and knowledgeably administer prescribed medications and treatments to patients with cardiac disorders.
6. Actively participate in planning and coordinating interprofesional care for patients with cardiac disorders.
7. Provide appropriate teaching and community-based care for patients with cardiac disorders and their families.
8. Evaluate the effectiveness of nursing care, revising the plan of care as needed to promote, maintain, or restore the functional health status of patients with cardiac disorders.

TERMS MATCHING

Place the letter of the correct definition in the space next to each term.

1. _____ aortic valve
2. _____ cardiac tamponade
3. _____ cardiomyopathy
4. _____ endocarditis
5. _____ heart failure
6. _____ hemodynamics
7. _____ mean arterial pressure (MAP)
8. _____ mitral valve
9. _____ murmur
10. _____ myocarditis
11. _____ orthopnea
12. _____ paroxysmal nocturnal dyspnea
13. _____ pericarditis
14. _____ pulmonary edema
15. _____ pulmonic valve
16. _____ regurgitation
17. _____ rheumatic fever
18. _____ rheumatic heart disease
19. _____ stenosis
20. _____ tricuspid valve
21. _____ valvular heart disease

A. A valve of the heart that lies between the left atrium and the left ventricle

B. This occurs when the valve fails to close properly, allowing blood to flow back through it

C. Compression of the heart due to pericardial effusion, trauma, cardiac rupture, or hemorrhage

D. The average pressure in the arterial circulation throughout the cardiac cycle; an indicator of tissue perfusion

E. The patient awakens at night acutely short of breath

F. A valve of the heart that lies between the right ventricle and the pulmonary artery

G. Interference of blood flow to, within, and from the heart

H. Primary abnormality of the heart muscle that affects its structural or functional characteristics

I. A valve of the heart located between the right atrium and the right ventricle

J. An abnormal accumulation of fluid in the interstitial tissue and alveoli of the lung

K. The study of forces involved in blood circulation

L. Condition where valve leaflets fuse together and are unable to open or close fully

M. A slowly progressive valvular deformity that may follow acute or repeated attacks of rheumatic fever

N. Inflammation of the endocardium

O. Inflammation of the pericardium

P. A systemic inflammatory disease caused by an abnormal immune response to pharyngeal infection by group A beta-hemolytic streptococci

Q. Inflammation of the heart muscle

R. Patient experiences difficulty breathing while lying down

S. The valve that lies between the left ventricle and the aorta

T. The most common cardiac disorder; the heart is unable to pump enough blood to meet the metabolic demands of the body

U. A sound associated with turbulent blood flow through the heart

FOCUSED STUDY

1. Describe the four stages of heart failure.

_____

_____

_____

_____

_____

2. Discuss the differences between acute and subacute infective endocarditis.

_____

_____

_____

_____

3. Discuss the different causes and clinical manifestations associated with dilated, hypertrophic, and restrictive cardiomyopathies.

_____

_____

_____

_____

_____

4. Explain the nursing responsibilities associated with administering positive inotropic agents.

_____

_____

_____

_____

CASE STUDY

James Hacking is a 76-year-old patient who has been admitted to the hospital with left-sided heart failure. A student nurse is observing the nurse care for Mr. Hacking. The student nurse asks the following questions about Mr. Hacking's condition.

1. What is heart failure?

2. What are the causes of heart failure?

3. What are some clinical manifestations associated with left-sided heart failure?

4. What are the complications of heart failure?

5. How is heart failure diagnosed?

6. Mr. Hacking's physician states that she wants a Swan-Ganz catheter to be placed. The student nurse requests information about this catheter and an explanation as to how it can be used to monitor Mr. Hacking's condition.

7. Mr. Hacking's physician writes an order for the nurse to administer fosinopril (Monopril®). The student nurse requests information about what type of medication this is and how it works.

CARE PLAN CRITICAL-THINKING ACTIVITY

Please refer to the case study and nursing care plan exercise A Patient with Heart Failure in your textbook to answer the following questions.

1. Why is it important for Ms. Snow to keep a record of symptoms and their frequency for 1 month?

2. List two drinks or food items that contain caffeine.

3. What is a complication of mitral valve prolapse about which Ms. Snow should be educated?

CROSSWORD PUZZLE

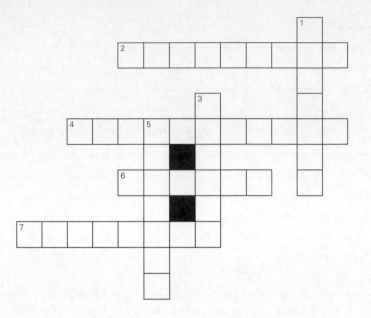

Across

2 The force needed to eject blood into the circulation

4 When the _____ nervous system is stimulated, the heart rate and contractility increase.

6 The amount of blood that returns to the ventricles

7 The ventricular filling time

Down

1 The ability of the heart to increase cardiac output to meet demand is the _____ reserve.

3 The volume of blood ejected with each heartbeat is the _____ volume.

5 The volume of blood in the ventricles prior to contraction

REVIEW QUESTIONS

1. A new nurse is providing education about prosthetic heart valves to a patient. What characteristic is considered an advantage of a prosthetic heart valve?
   1. long-term durability
   2. low incidence of thromboembolism
   3. no need for long-term anticoagulation
   4. quietness

2. During discharge planning, the nurse is teaching the patient with heart failure about home activity guidelines. What instruction is correct?
   1. "Eat three large meals each day."
   2. "It is okay to lift heavy objects."
   3. "Eat a low-fiber diet and restrict fluid intake."
   4. "Begin a graded exercise program."

3. A nurse is evaluating a patient's understanding about managing valvular disease. Which patient statement indicates the need for further teaching?
   1. "I will notify all of my healthcare providers about my valve disease."
   2. "I should have adequate rest to prevent fatigue."
   3. "I need to call my healthcare provider if I think I'm bleeding anywhere."
   4. "I will follow the diet restrictions to increase my body's ability to retain fluid."

4. The nurse is preparing to educate the patient about how to reduce the risk factors associated with heart failure. Which nursing intervention would be an unexpected addition to the patient's plan of care?

   1. Teach about coronary heart disease, which is a primary cause of heart failure.
   2. Stress the relationship between effective management of cirrhosis and reduced risk of heart failure.
   3. Discuss the importance of monitoring weight daily.
   4. Discuss the importance of taking antihypertensive medications as ordered to reduce the risk for heart failure.

5. A nurse is providing an educational seminar about pulmonary edema for nurses who work in the intensive care unit. What statement from one of the participants demonstrates the need for further education?

   1. "In cardiogenic pulmonary edema, the contractility of the right ventricle is severely impaired."
   2. "Pulmonary edema is a medical emergency."
   3. "Immediate treatment for acute pulmonary edema focuses on restoring effective gas exchange and reducing fluid and pressure in the pulmonary vascular system."
   4. "The patient often is restless and highly anxious, although severe hypoxia may cause confusion or lethargy."

6. Which statement by a student nurse reflects the needs for further education regarding rheumatic fever and rheumatic heart disease?

   1. "Rheumatic heart disease frequently damages the heart valves and is a major cause of mitral and aortic valve disorders."
   2. "Rheumatic fever is a systemic inflammatory disease caused by an abnormal immune response to pharyngeal infection by group A beta-hemolytic streptococci."
   3. "The peak incidence of rheumatic fever is in patients aged 22 to 35."
   4. "Rheumatic fever and rheumatic heart disease remain significant public health problems in many developing countries."

32

Nursing Care of Patients with **Vascular** and **Lymphatic Disorders**

LEARNING OUTCOMES

1. Compare and contrast the manifestations and effects of disorders affecting large and small vessels, arteries, and veins.
2. Explain risk factors for and measures to prevent peripheral vascular disorders and their complications.
3. Explain the nursing implications for medications and other interprofessional treatments used for patients with peripheral vascular disorders.
4. Describe preoperative and postoperative nursing care of patients having vascular surgery.
5. Relate the manifestations and diagnostic test results to the etiology and pathophysiology of common peripheral vascular and lymphatic disorders.

CLINICAL COMPETENCIES

1. Assess patients with peripheral vascular disorders, using data to select and prioritize appropriate nursing diagnoses and identify desired outcomes of care.
2. Identify the effects of peripheral vascular disorders on the functional health status of assigned patients.
3. Use research and an evidence-based plan to provide individualized care for patients with peripheral vascular disorders.
4. Collaborate with the interprofessional care team in planning and providing care for patients with peripheral vascular disorders.
5. Safely and knowledgably administer medications and prescribed treatments for patients with peripheral vascular disorders.
6. Provide patient and family teaching to promote, maintain, and restore health in patients with common peripheral vascular disorders.

TERMS MATCHING

Place the letter of the correct definition in the space next to each term.

1. _____ aneurysm
2. _____ atherosclerosis
3. _____ blood pressure (BP)
4. _____ chronic venous insufficiency
5. _____ deep venous thrombosis (DVT)
6. _____ diastolic blood pressure
7. _____ dissection
8. _____ embolism
9. _____ hypertension
10. _____ intermittent claudication
11. _____ lymphedema
12. _____ mean arterial pressure (MAP)
13. _____ peripheral vascular disease (PVD)
14. _____ primary hypertension
15. _____ pulse pressure
16. _____ Raynaud's disease/phenomenon
17. _____ secondary hypertension
18. _____ systolic blood pressure
19. _____ thromboangiitis obliterans
20. _____ thromboembolus
21. _____ thrombus
22. _____ varicose veins
23. _____ vasoconstriction
24. _____ vasodilation
25. _____ venous thrombosis

A. An occlusive vascular disease in which small and midsize peripheral arteries become inflamed and spastic, which causes clots to form; also called Buerger's disease

B. Irregular, tortuous veins with incompetent valves

C. An abnormal dilation of a blood vessel, commonly at a site of a weakness or tear in the vessel wall

D. Narrowing of the vessel lumen

E. A form of arteriosclerosis in which deposits of fat and fibrin obstruct and harden the arteries

F. The tension or pressure exerted by blood against arterial walls

G. Disorders characterized by episodes of intense vasospasm in the small arteries and arterioles of the fingers and sometimes the toes

H. A disorder of inadequate venous return over a prolonged period

I. Impaired blood supply to peripheral tissues, particularly the lower extremities

J. The sudden obstruction of a blood vessel by a clot or debris

K. Expansion of a vessel

L. An elevated blood pressure that results from an identifiable underlying process

M. A tear in the intima of the aorta with hemorrhage into the media

N. This can be calculated by subtracting the diastolic blood pressure from the systolic blood pressure

O. The minimum pressure maintained by elastic arterial walls during diastole (cardiac relaxation) to maintain blood flow through capillary beds

P. The average pressure in the arterial circulation throughout the cardiac cycle

Q. The sudden obstruction of a blood vessel by a thrombus

R. Cramping or pain in the leg muscles brought on by exercise and relieved by rest

S. The arterial pressure wave produced by ventricular contraction (systole)

T. A persistently elevated systemic blood pressure; also known as essential hypertension

U. Excess pressure in the arterial portion of systemic circulation

V. A disorder characterized by extremity edema due to accumulation of lymph

W. A condition in which a blood clot forms on the wall of a vein, accompanied by inflammation of the vein wall and some degree of obstructed venous blood flow; also known as thrombophlebitis

X. Blood clot (thrombus) formation and inflammation within a deep vein, usually in the pelvis or lower extremities; a common complication of hospitalization, surgery, and immobilization

Y. A blood clot

FOCUSED STUDY

1. Discuss the complex interactions and factors that result in primary hypertension.

_____

_____

_____

_____

2. Identify the ways that varicose veins can be diagnosed.

_____

_____

_____

_____

_____

3. Explain the nursing interventions that should be included in the plan of care for a patient who has developed fluid volume excess associated with lymphedema.

_____

_____

_____

4. Describe the clinical manifestations associated with progressive lymphedema.

_____

_____

_____

_____

_____

CASE STUDIES

Case Study 1

Josh Bradley is a 32-year-old patient who was admitted to the hospital yesterday with a hypertensive emergency. He tells the nurse that his physician was in early this morning and told him something about an arterial blood pressure, PVR, and MAP, but he can't remember what the physician said about each of them. Answer the following questions based on your knowledge of caring for a patient with a vascular disorder.

1. What factors influence arterial blood pressure?

2. Explain peripheral vascular resistance (PVR) and mean arterial pressure (MAP).

3. What are some common clinical manifestations found in patients experiencing hypertensive emergencies?

Case Study 2

Elizabeth Drake is a 44-year-old female patient who is visiting her physician's office to have her blood pressure checked. She is 5'5" and weighs 125 pounds. She states that she currently smokes one pack of cigarettes per day and drinks alcohol socially. The physician diagnoses her with primary hypertension. Answer the following questions based on your knowledge of caring for a patient with primary hypertension.

1. Discuss the manifestations of primary hypertension.

2. Explain the complications of primary hypertension.

3. Briefly summarize the lifestyle changes Ms. Drake should enact to help control her hypertension.

SHORT ANSWERS

Fill in the information regarding arterial ulcers and venous ulcers.

Factor	Arterial Ulcers	Venous Ulcers
Location		
Ulcer appearance		
Skin appearance		
Skin temperature		
Edema		
Pain		
Gangrene		
Pulses		

REVIEW QUESTIONS

1. Which pressure is felt as the peripheral pulse and heard as Korotkoff's sounds during blood pressure measurement?
   1. diastolic blood pressure
   2. systolic blood pressure
   3. pulse pressure
   4. mean arterial pressure

2. The nursing instructor asks the student nurse to provide the formula used to calculate the MAP. What formula should the student nurse provide for the instructor?
   1. [diastolic BP + 2 (systolic BP)] / 2
   2. [systolic BP + 2 (diastolic BP)] / 2
   3. [systolic BP + 2 (diastolic BP)] / 3
   4. [diastolic BP + 2 (systolic BP)] / 3

3. The nurse is implementing nursing interventions that can be used to reduce the risk of aneurysm rupture. Which strategy would be an unexpected addition to the patient's care plan?
   1. Maintain bed rest with legs elevated.
   2. Maintain a calm environment and implement measures to reduce psychologic stress.
   3. Instruct patient to prevent straining during defecation and to avoid holding his or her breath while moving.
   4. Administer beta blockers and antihypertensives as prescribed.

4. Which statement by a student nurse reflects an adequate understanding of Raynaud's disease?
   1. "The disease affects primarily older women between the ages of 60 and 80."
   2. "It is characterized by episodes of intense vasospasm in the small veins of the fingers and sometimes the toes."
   3. "It has no identifiable cause."
   4. "It has been called the 'red-yellow-white' disease."

5. A nurse is planning an educational program about varicose veins. Which statement is correct?
   1. "Elastic stockings should be removed eight times a day for 15 minutes."
   2. "Complications of varicose veins include venous insufficiency and stasis ulcers."
   3. "Prolonged sitting, the force of gravity, lack of leg exercise, and incompetent venous valves all weaken the muscle-pumping mechanism, which reduces arteriole blood return to the heart."
   4. "Varicose veins may be asymptomatic, but most cause manifestations such as severe aching leg pain, leg spasms, leg lightness, itching, or feelings of coldness in the legs."

6. During discharge planning, the nurse is teaching the patient about factors that contribute to hypertension. Which risk factor is considered to be modifiable?
   1. obesity
   2. age
   3. race
   4. family history

7. The patient has been diagnosed with lymphangitis. Which statement by the patient indicates an adequate understanding about this condition?
   1. "I just have some enlarged lymph nodes."
   2. "These red streaks and my fever are related to an infection."
   3. "The lymphangiography for which I'm scheduled can also be curative."
   4. "I really need to drink more fluids."

Nursing Care of Patients with **Hematologic Disorders**

LEARNING OUTCOMES

1. Relate the physiology and assessment of the hematologic system and related systems to commonly occurring hematologic disorders.
2. Describe the pathophysiology of common hematologic disorders.
3. Explain nursing implications for medications and other treatments prescribed for hematologic disorders.
4. Discuss indications for and complications of bone marrow or stem cell transplantation, as well as related nursing care.
5. Compare and contrast the pathophysiology, manifestations, and management of bleeding disorders.
6. Describe the major types of leukemia and the most common treatment modalities and nursing interventions.
7. Differentiate Hodgkin's disease from non-Hodgkin's lymphomas.

CLINICAL COMPETENCIES

1. Assess the effects of hematologic disorders and prescribed treatments on patients' functional health status.
2. Monitor and document continuing assessment data, including laboratory test results, subjective and objective information, and reporting data outside the normal or expected range.
3. Based on knowledge of pathophysiology, prescribed treatment, and assessed data, identify and prioritize nursing diagnoses for patients with hematologic disorders.
4. Use nursing research and evidence-based practice to identify and implement individualized nursing interventions for the patient with a hematologic disorder.
5. Safely administer prescribed medications and treatments for patients with hematologic disorders.
6. Collaborate with the interprofessional care team to plan and provide coordinated, effective care for patients with hematologic disorders.
7. Provide appropriate teaching for patients with hematologic disorders, evaluating learning and the need for continued reinforcement of information.
8. Use continuing assessment data to revise the plan of care as needed to restore, maintain, or promote functional health in the patient with a hematologic disorder.

TERMS MATCHING

Place the letter of the correct definition in the space next to each term.

1. _____ anemia
2. _____ aplastic anemia
3. _____ bone marrow transplant (BMT)
4. _____ disseminated intravascular coagulation (DIC)
5. _____ hemolytic anemia
6. _____ hemophilia
7. _____ hemostasis
8. _____ iron-deficiency anemia
9. _____ leukemia
10. _____ lymphoma
11. _____ multiple myeloma
12. _____ myelodysplastic syndrome (MDS)
13. _____ pernicious anemia
14. _____ polycythemia
15. _____ sickle cell crisis
16. _____ sickle cell disease
17. _____ stem cell transplant (SCT)
18. _____ thalassemia
19. _____ thrombocytopenia

A. A group of hereditary clotting factor disorders that lead to persistent and sometimes severe bleeding

B. A malignancy in which plasma cells multiply uncontrollably and infiltrate the bone marrow, lymph nodes, spleen, and other tissues

C. A condition manifested by failure of the bone marrow to produce all three types of blood cells

D. An alternative to a bone marrow transplant; results in complete and sustained replacement of the recipient's blood cell lines with cells derived from the donor stem cells

E. Bone marrow is infused through a central venous line into the patient

F. An excess of red blood cells characterized by a hematocrit higher than 55%; also known as erythrocytosis

G. Inherited disorders of hemoglobin synthesis in which the alpha or beta chain of the hemoglobin molecule is missing or defective

H. The ability of the body to control bleeding

I. Failure to absorb adequate amounts of vitamin B_{12}

J. A disruption of hemostasis characterized by widespread intravascular clotting and bleeding

K. A platelet count of less than 100,000 per milliliter of blood

L. The most common type of anemia; often caused by poor nutritional intake

M. Occurs in the patient who has sickle cell anemia; characterized by severe episodes of fever and intense pain

N. A malignancy of lymphoid tissue

O. A group of blood disorders characterized by abnormal-appearing bone marrow and cytopenia; it is not a single disease

P. A group of chronic malignant disorders of white blood cells and WBC precursors

Q. A hereditary, chronic hemolytic anemia; characterized by episodes of sickling

R. A condition that is characterized by premature destruction of red blood cells

S. An abnormally low number of circulating RBCs, hemoglobin concentration, or both

FOCUSED STUDY

1. List the names of some medications used to replace iron and treat iron-deficiency anemia. Briefly describe information the nurse should provide the patient who is receiving one of these medications.

   _____

   _____

   _____

2. List some clinical manifestations associated with polycythemia.

   _____

   _____

   _____

   _____

3. List some clinical manifestations associated with disseminated intravascular coagulation.

_____

_____

_____

_____

_____

4. Describe the differences between Hodgkin's disease and non-Hodgkin's lymphoma.

_____

_____

_____

_____

_____

CASE STUDY

Jonathan Obermark is a 13-year-old male patient who was diagnosed today with acute lymphoblastic leukemia (ALL). His mother was recently diagnosed with iron-deficiency anemia. Jonathan and his mother have some questions for the nurse and physician regarding these two conditions. Answer the following questions based on your knowledge of anemias and ALL.

1. What are the different types of anemias?

2. What are some dietary sources of heme and nonheme iron?

3. What are some common causes of iron-deficiency anemia?

4. Which population is most at risk for developing acute lymphoblastic leukemia (ALL)?

5. What are the associated clinical manifestations of ALL?

6. Jonathan has been scheduled for a chest x-ray to rule out pneumonia. How may pneumonia be related to ALL?

7. The nurse studies Jonathan's laboratory results and determines that his platelet count is low. What problems may arise because of this?

8. The physician spoke with Jonathan and his mother about how ALL is treated. Which medications are typically used?

CARE PLAN CRITICAL-THINKING ACTIVITY

Please refer to the case study and nursing care plan exercise A Patient with Hemophilia in your textbook to answer the following questions.

1. Why were an ice bag and manual pressure applied to Mr. Cruise's nose in the emergency department?

2. Why is it important for Mr. Cruise to avoid contact sports?

3. What information is available on a medical alert bracelet?

SHORT ANSWERS

List three conditions that may result in disseminated intravascular coagulation (DIC).

Tissue Damage	Vessel Damage	Infections
1.	1.	1.
2.	2.	2.
3.	3.	3.

REVIEW QUESTIONS

1. Which statement by a student nurse reflects an adequate understanding about iron-deficiency anemia?
    1. "Iron-deficiency anemia is the least common type of anemia."
    2. "The body can synthesize hemoglobin even without iron."
    3. "Inadequate dietary iron intake also contributes to anemia in the older adult."
    4. "Iron-deficiency anemia results in increased numbers of RBCs."

2. During discharge planning, the nurse is teaching the patient about the sources of heme iron. Which food is a source of nonheme iron?
    1. veal
    2. clams
    3. egg yolk
    4. dried fruits

3. The spouse of a patient who has leukemia is providing care for the patient at home. Which activity plan indicates the spouse's need for further teaching?
    1. Provide rest periods before meals.
    2. Provide prescribed medications for pain or nausea 10 minutes before meals.
    3. Provide liquids with different textures and tastes.
    4. Provide mouth care before and after meals.

4. The Ann Arbor Staging System is used to assess the extent and severity of lymphomas. Which stage is used to describe the patient who has involvement of lymph node regions or structures on both sides of the diaphragm?
    1. stage I
    2. stage II
    3. stage III
    4. stage IV

5. During discharge planning, the nurse is teaching the patient how to prevent or relieve nausea or vomiting. Which instruction would be unexpected?
    1. Eat soda crackers.
    2. Avoid unpleasant odors and get fresh air.
    3. Eat warm, spicy foods.
    4. Suck on hard candy.

6. A nurse is preparing an educational seminar about aplastic anemia. Which statement should not be included because it is inaccurate?
    1. "Manifestations of aplastic anemia include fatigue, pallor, progressive weakness, exertional dyspnea, headache, and ultimately tachycardia and heart failure."
    2. "In aplastic anemia, the bone marrow fails to produce red blood cells and platelets, but white cells are abundant."
    3. "Aplastic anemia may occur with viral infections such as mononucleosis, hepatitis C, and HIV disease."
    4. "Aplastic anemia is rare."

7. Which statement by a student nurse reflects an adequate understanding about polycythemia?
    1. "In primary polycythemia, RBC production is decreased."
    2. "Secondary polycythemia occurs when erythropoietin levels are elevated."
    3. "In relative polycythemia, the total RBC count is high."
    4. "In relative polycythemia, the hematocrit is abnormally low."

8. The patient has been diagnosed with acute lymphocytic leukemia. Which nursing intervention would be unexpected?
    1. Encourage visitors to visit with the patient to help provide emotional support.
    2. Provide oral hygiene after every meal.
    3. Ensure meticulous handwashing among all people who come in contact with the patient.
    4. Maintain protective isolation as indicated.

LEARNING OUTCOMES

1. Describe the anatomy, physiology, and functions of the respiratory system.
2. Compare and contrast factors affecting respiration.
3. Identify specific topics for consideration during a health history interview of the patient with health problems involving the respiratory system.
4. Give examples of genetic disorders of the respiratory system.
5. Describe normal variations in assessment findings for the older adult.
6. Identify abnormal findings that may indicate alterations in respiratory function.

CLINICAL COMPETENCIES

1. Complete a health history of the respiratory system, incorporating appraisal of physiological and psychosocial issues.
2. Conduct and document a health history for patients having or at risk for alterations in the respiratory system.
3. Conduct and document a physical assessment of respiratory structures and functions, demonstrating sensitivity and respect for the diversity of the human experience.
4. Monitor the results of diagnostic tests and communicate abnormal findings within the interprofessional team.

TERMS MATCHING

Place the letter of the correct definition in the space next to each term.

1. _____ apnea

2. _____ atelectasis

3. _____ bradypnea

4. _____ crackles

5. _____ friction rub

6. _____ lung compliance

7. _____ oxyhemoglobin

8. _____ surfactant

9. _____ tachypnea

10. _____ tidal volume (TV)

11. _____ vital capacity (VC)

12. _____ wheezes

A. The combination of oxygen and hemoglobin in arterial blood

B. The sound heard when two dry surfaces are rubbed together; auscultated during lung assessment

C. The collapse of lung tissue following obstruction of the bronchus or bronchioles

D. The volume inhaled and exhaled with normal quiet breathing

E. An abnormally slow respiratory rate

F. Continuous, musical sounds caused by narrowing of the lumen in a respiratory passage

G. An abnormally fast respiratory rate

H. A lipoprotein produced by the alveolar cells that interferes with the adhesion of water molecules, reducing surface tension and helping to expand the lungs

I. The ability of the lungs to distend under pressure

J. The total amount of air that can be exhaled after a maximal inspiration

K. Discontinuous lung sounds heard by auscultation; can be fine or coarse. Produced by air passing over airway secretions or the opening of collapsed airways

L. Cessation of breathing lasting from a few seconds to a few minutes

FOCUSED STUDY

1. Identify the functions of the pharynx and the larynx.

_____

_____

_____

_____

2. List at least two disorders of the respiratory system that have genetic influences.

_____

_____

3. List three age-related changes that occur in the respiratory system and the significance of each change.

_____

_____

_____

4. Describe the purpose of a bronchoscopy and the associated nursing interventions.

_____

_____

_____

_____

CASE STUDY

Drake Strattman has been working as a registered nurse for 11 years. He is the nursing manager of a unit in a local hospital that admits many patients with respiratory disorders. He has been asked to teach a class to nurses at the hospital today about the respiratory system and respiratory disorders. Answer the following questions based on your understanding of the respiratory system.

1. What are some factors that affect ventilation and respiration?

2. Where are the sinuses, and what is the purpose of sinuses?

3. What is the difference between inspiratory reserve volume (IRV) and expiratory reserve volume (ERV)?

4. What are some implications of changes in the patient's breathing pattern?

5. What are the different characteristics of vesicular, bronchovesicular, and bronchial breath sounds?

6. How does the patient's trachea location change when the patient has a pleural effusion, pneumothorax, or atelectasis?

SHORT ANSWERS

1. Identify the following structures: bronchi, bronchioles, alveolar ducts, and alveoli. Then compare your answers with Figure 34-3 on page 1067 of your textbook.

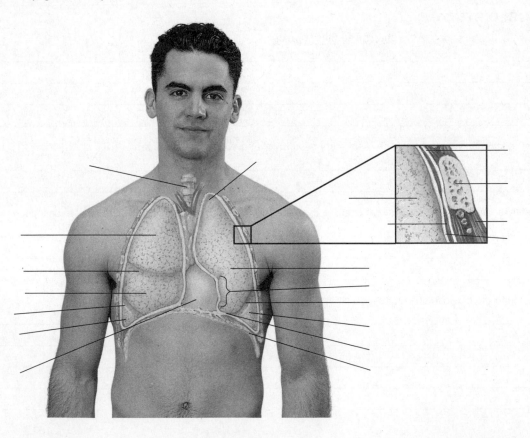

2. Fill in the labels for the blanks in the figure. Then compare your answers with Figure 34-4 on page 1068 of your textbook.

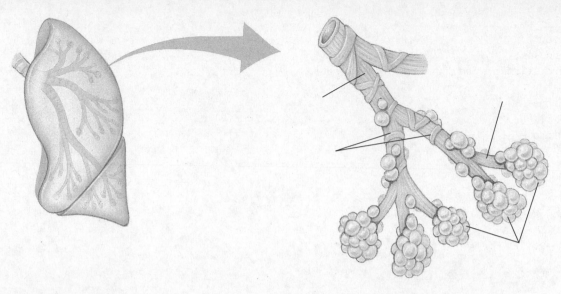

REVIEW QUESTIONS

1. A nurse is planning an educational program about the respiratory system. Which statement in the nurse's speaking notes should be corrected?
   1. "The laryngopharynx extends from the hyoid bone to the larynx."
   2. "The right lung is smaller and has two lobes, whereas the left lung has three lobes."
   3. "The parietal pleura lines the thoracic wall and mediastinum."
   4. "During expiration, carbon dioxide is expelled."

2. A nurse is evaluating a nursing student's understanding of inspiration and expiration. What statement indicates the need for further education?
   1. "During inspiration, the diaphragm contracts and flattens out to increase the vertical diameter of the thoracic cavity."
   2. "Expiration is primarily a passive process that occurs as a result of the elasticity of the lungs."
   3. "During expiration, the inspiratory muscles contract, the diaphragm descends, the ribs expand, and the lungs recoil."
   4. "A single inspiration lasts for about 1–1.5 seconds, whereas expiration lasts for about 2–3 seconds."

3. A nurse is evaluating a patient's understanding of some diagnostic tests that he had while in the hospital. Which statement by the patient indicates a need for further education?
   1. "Arterial blood gases are conducted to evaluate alterations in acid–base balances."
   2. "Pulse oximetry is used to evaluate or monitor the oxygen saturation of the blood."
   3. "A pulmonary angiography provides direct visualization of the larynx, trachea, and bronchi."
   4. "A thoracentesis, when done for diagnostic purposes, is conducted to obtain a specimen of pleural fluid."

4. Two nurses are discussing a patient's respiratory condition. Which statement by one of the nurses is correct?
   1. "Dullness is heard in patients with atelectasis, lobar pneumonia, and pleural effusion."
   2. "Retraction of intercostal spaces may be seen in pneumothorax."
   3. "Bulging of intercostal spaces may be seen in asthma."
   4. "Bilateral chest expansion is increased in emphysema."

5. Which structure is part of the lower respiratory tract?
   1. nose
   2. trachea
   3. pleura
   4. sinuses

6. Which structure is part of the upper respiratory tract?
   1. larynx
   2. lungs
   3. bronchi
   4. rib cage

Nursing Care of Patients with **Upper Respiratory Disorders**

LEARNING OUTCOMES

1. Relate the anatomy and physiology of the upper respiratory tract to commonly occurring disorders and risk factors for these disorders.
2. Describe the pathophysiology of common upper respiratory tract disorders, relating their manifestations to the pathophysiologic process.
3. Discuss nursing implications for medications and other interprofessional care measures to treat upper respiratory disorders.
4. Describe surgical procedures used to treat upper respiratory disorders and their implications for patient care and recovery.
5. Identify health promotion actitivities related to reducing the incidence of upper respiratory disorders, describing the appropriate population and setting for implementing the identified measures.
6. Discuss treatment options for oral and laryngeal cancers, along with their implications for the patient's body image and functional health.

CLINICAL COMPETENCIES

1. Assess the functional health status of patients with upper respiratory disorders, using data to identify and prioritize holistic nursing care needs.
2. Use nursing research and evidence-based practice to plan and implement nursing care for patients with upper respiratory disorders.
3. Provide safe and effective nursing care for patients having surgery involving the upper respiratory system and/or with a tracheostomy.
4. Safely administer medications and prescribed treatments for patients with disorders of the upper respiratory tract.
5. Provide appropriate teaching for the patient and family affected by upper respiratory tract disorders.
6. Evaluate the effectiveness of care, reassessing and modifying the plan of care as needed to achieve desired patient outcomes.

TERMS MATCHING

Place the letter of the correct definition in the space next to each term.

1. _____ coryza

2. _____ epistaxis

3. _____ influenza

4. _____ laryngectomy

5. _____ laryngitis

6. _____ pertussis

7. _____ pharyngitis

8. _____ rhinitis

9. _____ rhinoplasty

10. _____ sinusitis

11. _____ sleep apnea

12. _____ tonsillitis

A. Inflammation of the nasal cavities; the most common upper respiratory disorder

B. Acute inflammation of the pharynx

C. Profuse nasal discharge

D. A highly contagious acute upper respiratory infection caused by the bacterium *Bordetella pertussis*; also known as whooping cough

E. Surgical reconstruction of the nose

F. Surgical removal of the larynx

G. Inflammation of the mucous membranes of one or more of the sinuses

H. A nosebleed

I. Absence of airflow through the upper airways for 10 or more seconds

J. A highly contagious viral respiratory disease characterized by coryza, fever, cough, and systemic symptoms such as headache and malaise

K. Acute inflammation of the palatine tonsils

L. Inflammation of the larynx

FOCUSED STUDY

1. List four clinical manifestations associated with the common cold.

_____

_____

_____

2. List some common decongestants. Discuss health education that should be included for the patient who is taking decongestants.

_____

_____

_____

_____

_____

3. Discuss Reye's syndrome and how it relates to influenza.

_____

_____

_____

_____

4. Identify three risk factors associated with the development of laryngeal cancer.

_____

_____

_____

CASE STUDY

Nathaniel Smith is a 37-year-old male patient who has been diagnosed with obstructive sleep apnea. Part of the nursing responsibilities is to provide Nathaniel with education about sleep apnea before he leaves the clinic. Answer the following questions based on your knowledge of sleep apnea.

1. Explain the pathophysiology of sleep apnea.

2. List the manifestations of obstructive sleep apnea.

3. Review the risk factors associated with obstructive sleep apnea.

4. How is obstructive sleep apnea typically diagnosed?

5. Review the nonsurgical methods used to treat obstructive sleep apnea.

6. Review the surgical methods for treating obstructive sleep apnea.

7. Identify some common nursing diagnoses that may be used in the plan of care for Mr. Smith.

CARE PLAN CRITICAL-THINKING ACTIVITY

Please refer to the case study and nursing care plan exercise A Patient with Peritonsillar Abscess in your textbook to answer the following questions.

1. Why is it important for Ms. Wunderman to drink ice-cold fluids?

2. List the types of beverages and foods that Ms. Wunderman should avoid.

SHORT ANSWERS

Identify how laryngeal tumors are staged.

Stage 0	
Stage I	
Stage II	
Stage III	
Stage IV	

REVIEW QUESTIONS

1. A nurse is evaluating a patient's understanding of preventing the spread of an acute viral upper respiratory infection. Which patient statement indicates the need for further education?
   1. "I'll use tissues to cover my mouth and nose when I sneeze and cough so I won't spread my infection to other people."
   2. "I'll blow my nose with one nostril open to prevent infected matter from being forced into the eustachian tubes."
   3. "I'll wash my hands after I sneeze or cough."
   4. "I'll limit my use of nasal decongestants to prevent a rebound effect."
2. Which type(s) of influenza can be found in humans?
   1. A only
   2. A and C
   3. B and C
   4. A, B, and C

3. A nurse is teaching a patient about home care following a polypectomy. Which statement by the nurse is correct?
   1. "Apply hot compresses to the nose to decrease swelling, promote comfort, and prevent bleeding."
   2. "After nasal packing is removed, blow your nose every hour until clots are removed."
   3. "Avoid straining during bowel movements, vigorous coughing, and strenuous exercise."
   4. "Rest for 1 week after surgery to reduce the risk of bleeding."

4. A nurse is providing a patient's discharge teaching about tracheostomy stoma care and ways to prevent the development of respiratory infections. Which statement indicates that the nurse requires further education prior to providing this teaching?
   1. The patient may safely participate in water sports.
   2. The patient should increase fluid intake to maintain mucosal moisture and loosen secretions.
   3. The patient should shield the stoma with a stoma guard to prevent particulate matter from entering the lower respiratory tract.
   4. The patient should use a humidifier or vaporizer to add humidity to inspired air.

5. A nurse is planning an educational program about nasal polyps. Which statement in the nurse's speaking notes should be removed?
   1. "Polyps form in areas of dependent mucous membrane and present as pale, edematous masses that are covered with mucous membrane."
   2. "Nasal polyps are benign grapelike growths of the mucous membrane that lines the nose."
   3. "Polyps are unilateral and have a broad, firm base, which makes them rigid."
   4. "Polyps may be asymptomatic, although large polyps may cause nasal obstruction, rhinorrhea, and loss of sense of smell."

6. When discussing the management of sleep apnea with the nurse, the patient asks, "What are some methods I can use to manage my sleep apnea?" Which strategy should not be included?
   1. The nurse should discuss the relationship of alcohol and sedatives to sleep apnea and refer the patient to an alcohol treatment program or Alcoholics Anonymous as indicated.
   2. The nurse should recommend the use of the CPAP intermittently throughout the night.
   3. The nurse should discuss the relationship between obesity and sleep apnea.
   4. The nurse should recommend adequate fluid intake by the patient to maintain moist mucous membranes.

Nursing Care of Patients with **Ventilation Disorders**

LEARNING OUTCOMES

1. Relate the pathophysiology and manifestations of lower respiratory infections and inflammation, lung cancer, chest wall disorders, and trauma to the ability to maintain effective ventilation and respiration (gas exchange).

2. Compare and contrast the etiology, risk factors, and vulnerable populations for lower respiratory infections, lung cancer, chest wall disorders, and trauma.

3. Describe interprofessional care and the nursing role in health promotion and caring for patients with lower respiratory infections, lung cancer, chest wall disorders, and trauma.

4. Discuss surgery and other invasive procedures used to treat lung cancer, chest wall disorders, and trauma, and nursing responsibilities in caring for patients undergoing these procedures.

5. Describe the nursing implications for medications used to treat respiratory disorders and oxygen therapy.

CLINICAL COMPETENCIES

1. Assess the functional health status and the effects of lower respiratory and chest wall disorders on ventilation and gas exchange.

2. Use assessment data and knowledge of the effects of the disorder and prescribed treatment to identify priority nursing diagnoses and plan care for patients with lower respiratory disorders.

3. Use the nursing process and evidence-based nursing research to plan and implement individualized nursing care, including measures to promote ventilation and gas exchange, for patients with lower respiratory disorders.

4. Plan and provide appropriate teaching for health promotion among vulnerable populations and to prepare patients and families for continuity of care.

5. Evaluate the effectiveness of nursing interventions and teaching, revising strategies and teaching plans as needed.

6. Knowledgably and safely coordinate interprofessional care and administer prescribed medications and treatments for patients with lower respiratory disorders.

TERMS MATCHING

Place the letter of the correct definition in the space next to each term.

1. _____ asphyxiation
2. _____ bronchitis
3. _____ cyanosis
4. _____ dyspnea
5. _____ empyema
6. _____ flail chest
7. _____ hemoptysis
8. _____ hemothorax
9. _____ hypoxemia
10. _____ lung abscess
11. _____ pleural effusion
12. _____ pleuritis
13. _____ pneumonia
14. _____ pneumothorax
15. _____ severe acute respiratory syndrome (SARS)
16. _____ thoracentesis
17. _____ tuberculosis (TB)

A. Difficult or labored breathing
B. Low levels of oxygen in the blood
C. Inflammation of the pleura
D. The presence of blood in the pleural cavity
E. Inflammation of the respiratory bronchioles and alveoli
F. Oxygen deprivation
G. The accumulation of air in the pleural space
H. Bloody sputum
I. A lower respiratory illness; the infective agent is a type of coronavirus; first described in people in Asia in February 2003
J. The collection of excess fluid in the pleural space
K. When two or more consecutive ribs are fractured in multiple places, producing a free-floating segment of the chest wall
L. A gray, blue, or purple skin color that is caused by deoxygenated hemoglobin
M. A chronic, recurrent infectious disease that usually affects the lungs, although any organ can be affected; caused by *Mycobacterium tuberculosis*
N. An invasive procedure in which fluid or air is removed from the pleural space with a needle
O. An acute or chronic condition involving inflammation of the bronchi
P. An accumulation of purulent exudate in the pleural cavity
Q. A local area of necrosis and pus formation within the lung itself

FOCUSED STUDY

1. Discuss the nursing interventions that should be used for the patient with acute bronchitis.

_____

_____

_____

2. The lower respiratory tract is normally sterile. List the body's defense mechanisms used to maintain sterility in this area.

_____

_____

_____

_____

_____

3. Identify the clinical manifestations associated with a lung abscess.

_____

_____

_____

_____

4. Identify risk factors for developing tuberculosis.

_____

_____

_____

_____

CASE STUDY

Mimi Sutter is a 37-year-old female patient who is in the emergency department with complaints of shaking chills, fever, productive cough with yellow sputum, and pleuritic chest pain. The physician diagnoses her with acute bacterial pneumonia. Answer the following questions based on your knowledge of acute bacterial pneumonia.

1. What are some other clinical manifestations of acute bacterial pneumonia?

2. What are some differences in the way Ms. Sutter might present if she were older?

3. Ms. Sutter is diagnosed with pneumococcal pneumonia. What is the pathophysiology of this infection?

4. What are some diagnostic tests that were likely used to determine that Ms. Sutter has pneumococcal pneumonia?

5. Who should receive the pneumococcal pneumonia vaccine?

6. Who should not receive the influenza vaccine?

CARE PLAN CRITICAL-THINKING ACTIVITY

Please refer to the case study and nursing care plan exercise A Patient with Lung Cancer in your textbook to answer the following questions.

1. Mr. Mueller has small cell carcinoma. How might this disease affect Mr. Mueller's fluid balance?

2. What methods are available to assist Mr. Mueller to stop smoking?

SHORT ANSWERS

Fill in the blanks regarding the surgeries used to treat lung cancer.

Procedure	Description of Procedure	Used for
Laser bronchoscopy		
Mediastinoscopy		
Thoracotomy		
Wedge resection		
Segmental resection		
Sleeve resection (bronchoplastic reconstruction)		
Lobectomy		
Pneumonectomy		

REVIEW QUESTIONS

1. Which statement by a student nurse reflects an accurate understanding about pneumonia?
   1. "Inflammation of the bronchi is known as pneumonia."
   2. "Bacteria, viruses, fungi, protozoa, and other microbes can lead to infectious pneumonia."
   3. "Infectious causes of pneumonia include aspiration of gastric contents and inhalation of toxic or irritating gases."
   4. "The most common causative organism for community-acquired pneumonia is *Staphylococcus aureus*, a gram-negative bacterium."

2. Which statement regarding SARS is accurate?
   1. "The incubation period for SARS is generally 1 day."
   2. "A low-grade fever below 98.2°F is typically the initial manifestation of the disease."
   3. "The primary population affected by SARS is previously healthy children from 5 to 10 years of age."
   4. "The infective agent responsible for SARS is a coronavirus not previously identified in humans."

3. A nurse is preparing speaking notes for an educational program regarding tuberculosis. Which statement should be corrected prior to the presentation?
   1. "Primary or secondary tuberculosis lesions may affect other body systems such as the kidneys, the genitalia, bone, and the brain."
   2. "Worldwide, TB continues to be a significant health problem."
   3. "A previously healed tuberculosis lesion is unable to be reactivated."
   4. "*Mycobacterium tuberculosis* is a relatively slow-growing, slender, rod-shaped, acid-fast organism with a waxy outer capsule that increases its resistance to destruction."

4. A nurse is providing discharge teaching for the patient who has tuberculosis about some ways to prevent transmitting the disease to others. Which action by the patient indicates the need for further education?
   1. The patient always coughs and expectorates into tissues.
   2. The patient is placing the used tissues in a closed bag.
   3. The patient is wearing a mask when outside the negative air pressure room.
   4. The patient is using disposable silverware.

5. A nurse is evaluating a patient's understanding of histoplasmosis. Which statement by the patient indicates the need for further education?
   1. "The *Histoplasma capsulatum* organism is found in the soil and is linked to exposure to bird droppings and bats."
   2. "Initial chest x-rays are nonspecific; later ones show areas of calcification."
   3. "Histoplasmosis is the most common bacterial lung infection in the United States."
   4. "Infection occurs when the spores are inhaled and reach the alveoli."

6. A patient is scheduled for a thoracentesis. Which action by the nurse would be unexpected?
   1. Verify the presence of a signed informed consent for the procedure.
   2. Ensure that the patient has been fasting for 8–12 hours.
   3. Position the patient upright and leaning forward with the arms and head supported on an anchored overbed table.
   4. Administer a cough suppressant if indicated.

Nursing Care of Patients with Gas Exchange Disorders

37 CHAPTER

LEARNING OUTCOMES

1. Relate the pathophysiology and manifestations of obstructive, pulmonary vascular, and critical respiratory disorders to their effects on ventilation and respiration (gas exchange).
2. Compare and contrast the etiology, risk factors, and vulnerable populations for disorders affecting ventilation and gas exchange within the lungs.
3. Describe interprofessional care and the nursing role in health promotion and caring for patients with disorders that affect the ability to ventilate the lungs and exchange gases with the environment.
4. Discuss interprofessional interventions to provide airway and ventilatory support for the patient with respiratory failure, and nursing responsibilities in caring for patients who require airway and ventilatory support.
5. Describe the nursing implications for medications used to promote ventilation and gas exchange.

CLINICAL COMPETENCIES

1. Assess the functional health status of patients with disorders affecting ventilation and gas exchange.
2. Use assessment data and knowledge of the effects of a disorder and its prescribed treatment to identify priority nursing diagnoses and plan care for patients with disorders affecting ventilation and gas exchange.
3. Use the nursing process and evidence-based nursing research to plan and implement individualized nursing care for patients, including measures to promote ventilation and gas exchange.
4. Plan and provide appropriate teaching for health promotion among vulnerable populations and to prepare patients and families for continuity of care.
5. Evaluate the effectiveness of nursing interventions and teaching, revising strategies and teaching plans as needed.
6. Knowledgably and safely coordinate interprofessional care and administer prescribed medications and treatments for patients with disorders affecting ventilation and gas exchange.

TERMS MATCHING

Place the letter of the correct definition in the space next to each term.

1. _____ acute respiratory distress syndrome (ARDS)
2. _____ asthma
3. _____ atelectasis
4. _____ bronchiectasis
5. _____ chronic bronchitis
6. _____ chronic obstructive pulmonary disease (COPD)
7. _____ cor pulmonale
8. _____ cystic fibrosis (CF)
9. _____ emphysema
10. _____ pulmonary embolism
11. _____ pulmonary hypertension (PHTN)
12. _____ respiratory failure
13. _____ sarcoidosis
14. _____ status asthmaticus
15. _____ weaning

A. A chronic multisystem disease characterized by an exaggerated cellular immune response in involved tissues

B. A condition characterized by permanent abnormal dilation of one or more large bronchi and destruction of bronchial walls; initiated by inflammation, usually due to recurrent airway infections

C. A disorder characterized by noncardiac pulmonary edema and progressive refractory hypoxemia; also known as shock lung and adult hyaline membrane disease

D. A disorder of excessive bronchial mucus secretion; characterized by a productive cough lasting 3 or more months in two consecutive years

E. A chronic inflammatory disorder of the airways characterized by recurrent episodes of wheezing, breathlessness, chest tightness, and coughing

F. Severe, prolonged asthma that does not respond to routine treatment

G. The process of removing ventilator support and reestablishing spontaneous, independent respirations

H. Chronic airflow obstruction due to chronic bronchitis and/or emphysema

I. An abnormal elevation of the pulmonary arterial pressure

J. A condition associated with many respiratory disorders; a state of partial or total lung collapse and airlessness

K. An autosomal recessive disorder that affects epithelial cells of the respiratory, gastrointestinal, and reproductive tracts and leads to abnormal exocrine gland secretions

L. Inability of the lungs to oxygenate the blood and remove carbon dioxide adequately to meet the body's needs, even while resting

M. An obstruction of blood flow in part of the pulmonary vascular system by an embolus

N. A condition of right ventricular hypertrophy and failure resulting from long-standing pulmonary hypertension

O. A disorder characterized by destruction of the walls of the alveoli, with resulting enlargement of abnormal air spaces

FOCUSED STUDY

1. Identify two age-related changes of the pulmonary system.

   _____

   _____

   _____

   _____

2. Provide two examples of medications that are classified as methylxanthines. Identify clinical manifestations that may indicate that the patient has developed toxicity.

   _____

   _____

   _____

   _____

3. Identify the patient population that should be prescribed leukotriene modifiers. List three examples of medications that are classified as leukotriene modifiers.

_____

_____

_____

_____

_____

4. Explain how to perform pursed-lip breathing, diaphragmatic breathing, and coughing exercises.

_____

_____

_____

_____

CASE STUDY

Isabella Hitt is a 12-year-old patient who has been brought to the clinic by her mother, Anne. Isabella is coughing, wheezing, and stating that her chest hurts. Anne is very agitated and tells the nurse, "My daughter is having an asthma attack and needs an inhaler right away." Answer the following questions based on your knowledge of asthma.

1. Summarize the triggers of asthma.

2. List the clinical manifestations associated with acute asthma.

3. Explain how to use a metered-dose inhaler and a dry powder inhaler.

4. Discuss methods that can be used to prevent asthma attacks.

5. What is the underlying pathophysiology of asthma?

6. What is status asthmaticus?

7. What diagnostic tests can be used to diagnose asthma?

CARE PLAN CRITICAL-THINKING ACTIVITY

Please refer to the case study and nursing care plan exercise A Patient with ARDS in your textbook to answer the following question.

1. Why is it important to monitor Ms. Adamson's urine output hourly and to report output of less than 30 mL per hour?

SHORT ANSWERS

Fill in the blanks regarding the stepwise approach to asthma management in adults.

Step/Disease Severity	Preferred Treatment	Alternative or As-Needed Treatment
Step 1 Mild Intermittent		
Step 2 Mild Persistent		
Step 3 Moderate Persistent		
Step 4 Severe Persistent		

REVIEW QUESTIONS

1. Which set of clinical manifestations is an unexpected finding in a patient with cystic fibrosis?
   1. secretions in affected organs becoming very thin and runny
   2. excess mucus production in the respiratory tract impairing ability to clear secretions
   3. pancreatic enzyme deficiency that impairs digestion
   4. abnormal elevation of sodium and chloride concentrations in sweat

2. Which statement by a student nurse reflects an accurate understanding about atelectasis?
   1. "The least common cause of atelectasis is obstruction of the bronchus that ventilates a segment of lung tissue."
   2. "It is a state of partial or total lung collapse and airlessness."
   3. "It is a chronic condition."
   4. "The secondary therapy for atelectasis is prevention."

3. Which technique should the nurse teach a patient learning how to use a metered-dose inhaler with a spacer?
   1. Firmly insert a charged metered-dose inhaler canister into the device.
   2. Hold the canister upright, place the mouthpiece in the mouth, and close the lips around it.
   3. Press and hold the canister down while inhaling deeply and slowly for 8 to 10 seconds.
   4. Roll the canister between the palms, but do not vigorously shake the device.

4. A nurse is evaluating a patient's ability to use a dry powder inhaler. Which patient action indicates the need for further education?
   1. The patient removed the cap and held the inhaler upright.
   2. The patient held the inhaler level, with the mouthpiece end facing up.
   3. The patient removed the inhaler from his mouth and held his breath for 10 seconds.
   4. The patient exhaled slowly through pursed lips.

5. Which nursing intervention for a patient with chronic obstructive pulmonary disease (COPD) is correct?
   1. Restrict fluid intake to 1,500 mL per day.
   2. Elevate the head of the patient's bed no more than 15 degrees.
   3. Teach the "huff" coughing technique.
   4. Administer beclomethasone inhaler before ipratropium inhaler.

Assessing Patients with **Musculoskeletal Disorders**

LEARNING OUTCOMES

1. Describe the anatomy, physiology, and functions of the musculoskeletal system.
2. Identify specific topics for consideration during a health history interview of the patient with health problems involving the musculoskeletal system.
3. Describe normal variations in assessment findings for the older adult.
4. Give examples of genetic disorders of the musculoskeletal system.
5. Identify manifestations of impairment of the musculoskeletal system.

CLINICAL COMPETENCIES

1. Conduct and document a health history for patients who have or are at risk for alterations in the musculoskeletal system, eliciting patient values, preferences, and expressed needs as part of this interview.
2. Conduct and document a physical assessment of musculoskeletal structures and functions, demonstrating sensitivity and respect for the diversity of human experience.
3. Monitor the results of diagnostic tests and communicate abnormal findings within the interprofessional team.

TERMS MATCHING

Place the letter of the correct definition in the space next to each term.

1. _____ bursitis
2. _____ crepitation
3. _____ hematopoiesis
4. _____ kyphosis
5. _____ lordosis
6. _____ ossification
7. _____ osteoblast
8. _____ osteoclast
9. _____ scoliosis
10. _____ synovitis
11. _____ tendonitis

A. A lateral, S-shaped curvature of the spine
B. Blood cell formation
C. An increased lumbar curve
D. Inflammation of a bursa
E. The process of bone formation
F. Inflammation of the synovial membrane lining the articular capsule of a joint
G. A grating sound
H. Inflammation of a tendon
I. An exaggerated thoracic curvature of the spine common in older adults
J. Cells that resorb bone
K. Cells that form bone

FOCUSED STUDY

1. List manifestations of impairment of the musculoskeletal system.

_____

_____

_____

2. List specific topics for consideration during a health history interview of the patient with health problems that involve the musculoskeletal system.

_____

_____

_____

3. Summarize the anatomy, physiology, and functions of the musculoskeletal system.

_____

_____

_____

4. Describe the normal movements allowed by synovial joints.

_____

_____

_____

CASE STUDY

Michael Baldwin, RN, is preparing for a seminar about the musculoskeletal system. To assess the participants' understanding of the material he is presenting, Michael decides to develop a series of questions. Answer the following questions based on your knowledge of the musculoskeletal system.

1. Bones are classified by which shapes?

2. Summarize bone remodeling in adults.

3. What are the different types of joints as classified by function?

SHORT ANSWERS

Complete the chart regarding the structural classification of joints.

Type	Description	Examples
Fibrous		
Cartilaginous		
Synovial		

REVIEW QUESTIONS

1. A nurse is evaluating a patient's understanding of the musculoskeletal system. Which statement by the patient indicates a need for further teaching?
   1. "The musculoskeletal system is composed of bones, cartilage, ligaments, tendons, muscles, and joints."
   2. "The bones serve as a framework for the body and as a place for muscles, tendons, and ligaments to attach."
   3. "The musculoskeletal system allows both gross movement and fine movement."
   4. "The tissues and structures of the musculoskeletal system perform one function, which is movement."

2. Which statement about bones is false?
   1. Bones store minerals.
   2. The human skeleton is made up of 226 bones.
   3. Bones of the skeletal system are divided into the axial and the appendicular skeletons.
   4. Bones protect vital organs from injury.

3. Which type of bone has a midportion or a shaft?
   1. short
   2. long
   3. irregular
   4. flat

4. A patient who has a fracture in the wrist has likely fractured which type of bone?
   1. irregular
   2. long
   3. flat
   4. short

5. Which of the following is not a type of muscle tissue in the body?
   1. rough muscle
   2. skeletal muscle
   3. smooth muscle
   4. cardiac muscle

6. The body has approximately how many skeletal muscles?
   1. 200
   2. 400
   3. 600
   4. 800

7. Which type of joint is freely moveable, allows many kinds of movements, and is found at all articulations of the limbs?
   1. amphiarthrosis
   2. synarthroses
   3. fibrous
   4. synovial

8. During a patient assessment, what is the nurse likely to request of the patient to assess abduction?
    1. "Make a fist."
    2. "Turn your arm over at the elbow."
    3. "Spread your fingers."
    4. "Bend at the waist."

9. What is the term for a lateral, S-shaped curvature of the spine?
    1. lordosis
    2. scoliosis
    3. kyphosis
    4. synovitis

10. Numbness and burning in the fingers during which test may indicate carpal tunnel syndrome?
    1. bulge
    2. Thomas
    3. Phalen's
    4. McMurray's

Nursing Care of Patients with **Musculoskeletal Trauma**

LEARNING OUTCOMES

1. Compare and contrast the causes, risk factors, pathophysiology, manifestations, interprofessional care, and nursing care of contusions, strains, sprains, joint dislocations, and fractures.

2. Describe the pathophysiology, interprofesssional care, and nursing care for repetitive use injuries.

3. Describe the stages of bone healing.

4. Explain the pathophysiology, manifestations, and related treatment for complications of fractures: compartment syndrome, fat embolism syndrome, deep venous thrombosis, infection, delayed union and nonunion, and complex regional pain syndrome.

5. Discuss the purposes and related nursing interventions for casts, fixation devices, traction, and stump care.

6. Explain the causes, levels, types, and potential complications (infection, delayed healing, chronic stump pain, phantom pain, and contractures) of an amputation.

CLINICAL COMPETENCIES

1. Assess the health status of patients with musculoskeletal injuries, including the patient's perception of the injury, its impact on lifestyle, and expectations for care.

2. Use evidence-based research and guidelines to plan, coordinate, and implement care for patients who have experienced musculoskeletal trauma.

3. Determine priority nursing diagnoses, based on assessment data, to plan and implement individualized nursing interventions and teaching for patients with musculoskeletal injuries.

4. Provide skilled care for patients with a cast, fixation device, traction, or amputation, maintaining patient and caregiver safety at all times.

5. Coordinate and integrate interprofessional care into the care of patients with musculoskeletal trauma.

6. Communicate and document care for patients with traumatic injuries of the musculoskeletal system using electronic medical records and other communication methods as appropriate.

TERMS MATCHING

Place the letter of the correct definition in the space next to each term.

1. _____ amputation

2. _____ compartment syndrome

3. _____ contracture

4. _____ contusion

5. _____ dislocation

6. _____ fat embolism syndrome (FES)

7. _____ flail chest

8. _____ fracture

9. _____ phantom limb pain

10. _____ sprain

11. _____ strain

12. _____ subluxation

A. Bleeding into soft tissue resulting from a blunt force

B. An abnormal flexion and fixation of a joint caused by muscle atrophy and shortening

C. A stretch and/or tear of one or more ligaments surrounding a joint

D. A disorder characterized by neurologic dysfunction; pulmonary insufficiency; and a petechial rash on the chest, axilla, and upper arms

E. The partial or total removal of an extremity

F. The fracture of two or more adjacent ribs in two or more places and the formation of a free-floating segment that moves in the opposite direction of the rib cage

G. Excess pressure constricts the structures within a compartment and reduces circulation to muscles and nerves

H. A partial dislocation in which the bones of the joint remain in partial contact

I. Stretching or tearing of muscle fibers that results in bleeding into the tissues

J. Any break in the continuity of a bone

K. Separation of contact between two bones of a joint

L. A confusing pain syndrome that occurs following surgical or traumatic amputation of a limb

FOCUSED STUDY

1. Explain the interprofessional care and nursing care for repetitive use injuries: carpal tunnel syndrome, bursitis, and epicondylitis.

_____

_____

_____

_____

_____

2. Describe the nursing interventions for casts, traction, and internal fixation.

_____

_____

_____

_____

3. Summarize the stages of bone healing.

_____

_____

_____

4. List the potential complications of an amputation.

_____

_____

_____

CASE STUDY

Georgene Smith, a 12-year-old female patient, presented at the clinic after experiencing an injury while ice skating. Georgene states that she heard her right knee "pop" after she landed from an axle jump. Her knee is swollen with slight discoloration. Her pain assessment score is 9 out of 10. Answer the following questions based on your knowledge of sprains and strains.

1. Define *strain* and *sprain*.

2. Give examples of how a strain or sprain could occur.

3. What are the manifestations of a strain and a sprain?

4. Explain RICE therapy.

SHORT ANSWERS

Fill in the table regarding the manifestations of fractures.

Manifestation	Pathophysiology
	Abnormal position of bones secondary to fracture and muscles pulling on fractured bone
	Edema from localization of serous fluid and bleeding
	Muscle spasm, direct tissue trauma, nerve pressure, movement of fractured bone
	Nerve damage or nerve entrapment
	Pain
	Grating of bones or entrance of air into an open fracture
	Blood loss or associated injuries
	Muscle contraction near the fracture
	Extravasation of blood into the subcutaneous tissue

REVIEW QUESTIONS

1. Which statement about a strain is correct?
   1. The most common sites for a muscle strain are the wrist and ankle.
   2. The manifestations of a strain include pain, limited motion, muscle spasms, swelling, and possible muscle weakness.
   3. Severe strains that partially or completely tear the ligament are very painful but are not disabling.
   4. A strain is a stretch and/or tear of one or more ligaments that surround a joint.
2. What is the meaning of *R* in RICE therapy for musculoskeletal injuries?
   1. rest
   2. relax
   3. raise
   4. rub

3. Which injury has occurred when the ends of bones are forced from their normal position?
   1. dislocation
   2. strain
   3. sprain
   4. fracture

4. Which statement about fractures is correct?
   1. Fractures do not vary in severity.
   2. A fracture occurs when the bone is subjected to less kinetic energy than it can absorb.
   3. Not all of the 206 bones in the body can be fractured.
   4. Two basic mechanisms produce fractures: direct force and indirect force.

5. A nurse is evaluating a student's understanding of compartment syndrome. Which statement by the student indicates a need for further teaching?
   1. "Compartment syndrome usually develops within the first 24 hours of injury, when edema is at its peak."
   2. "Compartment syndrome occurs when excess pressure in a limited space constricts the structures in a compartment, which reduces circulation to muscles and nerves."
   3. "Acute compartment syndrome may result from hemorrhage and edema in the compartment after a fracture, from a crush injury, or from external compression of the limb by a cast that is too tight."
   4. "The fascia expands to support the muscles, nerves, and blood vessels of the extremities."

6. Which type of traction is the application of a pulling force through placement of pins into the bone?
   1. skin
   2. skeletal
   3. balanced suspension
   4. manual

7. Which statement by a student nurse reflects correct understanding about casts?
   1. "The cast is applied to immobilize the joint above and the joint below the fractured bone so that the bone will not move during healing."
   2. "A plaster cast may require up to 24 hours to dry, whereas a fiberglass cast dries in 2 hours."
   3. "Casts are applied on patients who have unstable fractures."
   4. "The cast must be allowed to partially dry before any pressure is applied to it."

8. During discharge planning, the nurse is teaching the patient about cast care. Which statement should be included in this teaching?
   1. "Scratch under a cast with a dull object."
   2. "Cover the cast while it is drying."
   3. "A cold sensation is normal during drying."
   4. "Use a blow dryer on the cool setting to relieve itching by blowing cool air into the cast."

9. Which instruction is incorrect for preserving an amputated part until it can be surgically reattached?
   1. Put the amputated part in direct contact with ice or water.
   2. Apply firm pressure to the bleeding area with a towel or an article of clothing.
   3. Send the amputated part to the emergency department with the injured person and make sure the emergency personnel know what it is.
   4. Wrap the amputated part in a clean cloth.

Nursing Care of Patients with **Musculoskeletal Disorders**

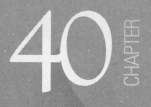

LEARNING OUTCOMES

1. Explain the etiology, pathophysiology, manifestations, complications, interprofessional care, and nursing care of musculoskeletal disorders.

2. Compare and contrast the pathophysiology, manifestations, diagnosis, and management of osteoporosis, osteoarthritis, Paget's disease, and rheumatoid arthritis.

3. Discuss the purposes, nursing implications, and health education for the patient and family for medications used to prevent and treat specific musculoskeletal disorders.

4. Describe the surgical procedures used to treat patients with arthritis.

CLINICAL COMPETENCIES

1. Assess the functional status of patients with musculoskeletal disorders, eliciting patient values, preferences, and expressed needs.

2. Use evidence-based research and practice guidelines to plan, provide, and manage safe and effective individualized care for patients with musculoskeletal disorders.

3. Determine priority nursing diagnoses, based on assessment data, to select and implement patient-centered nursing interventions for patients with musculoskeletal disorders.

4. Monitor patient responses to interprofessional and nursing interventions, recognizing, documenting, and reporting adverse or unanticipated responses.

5. Demonstrate effective use of strategies to reduce the risk of harm to patients with musculoskeletal disorders.

6. Integrate and coordinate interprofessional care into the care of patients with musculoskeletal disorders.

7. Use quality measures to identify gaps between local and best practices when caring for patients with musculoskeletal disorders.

8. Use the electronic medical record to plan, document care provided, and revise the plan of care as appropriate.

TERMS MATCHING

Place the letter of the correct definition in the space next to each term.

1. _____ arthritis

2. _____ arthroplasty

3. _____ arthroscopy

4. _____ fibromyalgia

5. _____ gout

6. _____ osteoarthritis (OA)

7. _____ osteomyelitis

8. _____ osteoporosis

9. _____ rheumatic disorders

10. _____ rheumatoid arthritis (RA)

11. _____ systemic lupus erythematosus (SLE)

12. _____ tophi

A. The reconstruction or replacement of a joint; may involve partial joint replacement or reshaping of the bones of a joint

B. Surgical procedure in which an arthroscope is inserted into a joint

C. Also called degenerative joint disease; characterized by loss of articular cartilage in articulating joints and hypertrophy of the bones at the articular margins

D. A metabolic disorder characterized by an acute inflammatory arthritis triggered by crystallization of urate in the joints

E. A chronic inflammatory autoimmune disease that affects almost all body systems, including the musculoskeletal system; characteristic manifestation is a red butterfly rash across the cheeks and bridge of the nose

F. A chronic systemic autoimmune disease that causes inflammation of connective tissue, primarily in the joints

G. Inflammation of the joints

H. Urate crystal deposits resulting from gout

I. A common rheumatic syndrome characterized by musculoskeletal pain, stiffness, and tenderness

J. Porous bones

K. Inflammatory diseases of connective tissues that affect joints, the muscles, and bones

L. Infection of the bone

FOCUSED STUDY

1. Discuss the surgical procedures used to treat patients with arthritis.

_____

_____

_____

2. Summarize the treatments for osteoporosis, osteoarthritis, Paget's disease, and rheumatoid arthritis.

_____

_____

_____

3. Describe the health education for the patient and family for medications used to treat osteoporosis, Paget's disease, gout, osteomalacia, osteoarthritis, rheumatoid arthritis, systemic lupus erythematosus, osteomyelitis, bone tumors, scleroderma, and low back pain.

_____

_____

_____

_____

_____

_____

_____

_____

_____

4. Briefly discuss treatments and diagnostics associated with muscular dystrophy (MD).

_____

_____

_____

_____

_____

_____

CASE STUDY

Christine Scott is a 37-year-old patient in today for her yearly physical. She tells the nurse that her mother was diagnosed with osteoporosis 2 weeks ago. Christine then asks a few questions. Answer her questions based on your knowledge of musculoskeletal disorders.

1. "What are the unmodifiable risk factors for osteoporosis?"

2. "What are the modifiable risk factors for osteoporosis?"

3. "What are the most common signs and symptoms of osteoporosis?"

4. "Will you explain any complications of osteoporosis?"

CARE PLAN CRITICAL-THINKING ACTIVITY

Please refer to the case study and nursing care plan exercise A Patient with Rheumatoid Arthritis in your textbook to answer the following questions.

1. Ms. James is diagnosed with rheumatoid arthritis at age 40. At what age does rheumatoid arthritis typically occur?

2. List the causes of rheumatoid arthritis.

3. Where can Ms. James obtain information about rheumatoid arthritis?

SHORT ANSWERS

Fill in the table differentiating between the features of osteoporosis and osteomalacia.

Differentiating Features	Osteoporosis	Osteomalacia
Pathophysiology		
Calcium level (serum)		
Phosphate level (serum)		
Parathyroid hormone level (serum)		
Alkaline phosphatase level (serum)		
Hydroxyproline (urine)		
Radiographic findings		

REVIEW QUESTIONS

1. During discharge planning, the nurse is teaching the patient about osteoporosis. Which information should the nurse include?
    1. Calcitonin (Miacalcin®) is a hormone that decreases bone formation and increases bone resorption.
    2. The most common manifestations of osteoporosis are loss of height; progressive curvature of the spine; low back pain; and fractures of the forearm, spine, or hip.
    3. Renal calculi are the most common complication of osteoporosis.
    4. Osteoporosis is not preventable or treatable.

2. Which statement by a student nurse reflects correct understanding about Paget's disease?
    1. "The most common manifestation of Paget's disease is localized pain of the short bones."
    2. "Paget's disease is a progressive metabolic skeletal disorder of the osteoclasts that results from excessive metabolic activity in bone, with excessive bone resorption followed by excessive bone formation."
    3. "The bones decrease in size and thickness in Paget's disease."
    4. "Paget's disease is also called osteoporosis."

3. A nurse is evaluating a nursing student's understanding of gout. Which statement by the nursing student indicates a need for further teaching?
    1. "Over time, urate deposits in subcutaneous tissues cause the formation of small white nodules called tophi."
    2. "Gout has an acute onset, usually at night, and often involves the fifth metatarsophalangeal joint."
    3. "Kidney disease may occur in patients with untreated gout, particularly when hypertension is present."
    4. "Serum uric acid is nearly always decreased in persons with gout."

4. A nurse is planning a seminar about osteomalacia. Which statement on a handout should be corrected?
    1. Hyperphosphatemia can result from insufficient dietary intake, excessive losses through the urine or stool, or a shift into the cells.
    2. The manifestations of osteomalacia include bone pain and tenderness.
    3. The primary causes of osteomalacia are calcium deficiency and hyperphosphatemia.
    4. Osteomalacia is a metabolic bone disorder characterized by inadequate or delayed mineralization of bone matrix in mature compact and spongy bone, which results in softening of bones.

5. A nurse is evaluating a nursing student's understanding of osteoarthritis. Which statement by the nursing student demonstrates a need for further teaching?
    1. "The onset of osteoarthritis (OA) is usually gradual and insidious, and the course is slowly progressive."
    2. "Osteoarthritis is the most common form of arthritis and is a leading cause of pain and disability in older adults."
    3. "Increasing age is the primary risk factor for OA."
    4. "Women are affected more often than men and at an earlier age, but the rate of osteoarthritis in men exceeds that of women by the middle adult years."

6. Which finding is not a manifestation of systemic lupus erythematosus (SLE)?
    1. unexplained fever
    2. white skin discoloration, especially on the face
    3. extreme fatigue
    4. painful or swollen joints

7. Hallux valgus is the enlargement and lateral displacement of the first metatarsal (the great toe). What is another word for *hallux valgus*?
    1. bunion
    2. hammertoe
    3. claw toe
    4. Morton's neuroma

8. Which condition is a lateral curvature of the spine?
    1. scoliosis
    2. kyphosis
    3. hunchback
    4. lordosis

Assessing the Nervous System

LEARNING OUTCOMES

1. Describe the anatomy, physiology, and functions of the nervous system.
2. Explain manifestations of impairment of neurologic function.
3. Give examples of genetic disorders of the nervous system.
4. Describe normal variations in assessment findings for the older adult.
5. Identify specific topics for consideration during a health history assessment interview of the patient with neurologic disorders.
6. Explain techniques for assessment of neurologic function.
7. Identify abnormal findings that may indicate alterations in nervous system function.

CLINICAL COMPETENCIES

1. Conduct and document a health history for patients having or at risk for alterations in the neurologic system.
2. Conduct and document a physical assessment of neurologic structures and functions, demonstrating sensitivity and respect for the diversity of the human experience.
3. Monitor the results of diagnostic tests and communicate abnormal findings within the interprofessional team.
4. Perform specific neurologic assessments for patients with suspected meningeal irritation and for patients who are disoriented or comatose.

TERMS MATCHING

Place the letter of the correct definition in the space next to each term.

1. _____ anosmia

2. _____ aphasia

3. _____ ataxia

4. _____ decerebrate posturing

5. _____ decorticate posturing

6. _____ diaphoresis

7. _____ dysarthria

8. _____ dysphagia

9. _____ dysphonia

10. _____ fasciculations

11. _____ flaccidity

12. _____ kinesthesia

13. _____ nystagmus

14. _____ ptosis

15. _____ spasticity

16. _____ tremors

A. Difficulty speaking

B. Drooping eyelids

C. Uncoordinated, irregular gait and muscle movement; weakness

D. Involuntary twitching or irregular movements

E. Increased muscle tone in disease of the corticospinal motor tract

F. An inability to smell

G. Abnormal posture resulting from lesions of the corticospinal tracts

H. The ability to assess movement or sense of position

I. Change in the tone of the voice

J. Rhythmic movements

K. Defective or absent language function

L. Abnormal posture resulting from lesions of the midbrain, pons, or diencephalon

M. Copious production of sweat

N. Decreased muscle tone

O. Involuntary eye movement

P. Difficulty swallowing

FOCUSED STUDY

1. What are the components of an abbreviated neurological assessment, or neuro check?

_____

_____

_____

_____

2. List specific topics to consider during a health history assessment interview of the patient with neurologic disorders.

_____

_____

_____

_____

_____

3. Discuss the anatomy, physiology, and functions of the nervous system.

_____

_____

_____

_____

_____

4. Discuss age-related changes in the nervous system.

_____

_____

_____

_____

_____

CASE STUDY

James Smith is a new nursing student who is attending a seminar about the central nervous system. At the end of the seminar, he asks a few questions. Answer his questions based on your knowledge of the central nervous system.

1. "What are the four major regions of the brain?"

2. "What components make up the diencephalon?"

3. "What are the purposes of cerebrospinal fluid?"

4. "How many pairs of spinal nerves are there, and where are they located?"

SHORT ANSWERS

Fill in the table regarding the functions of the cranial nerves.

Name	Function
I Olfactory	
II Optic	
III Oculomotor	
IV Trochlear	
V Trigeminal	
VI Abducens	
VII Facial	
VIII Acoustic	
IX Glossopharyngeal	
X Vagus	
XI Accessory	
XII Hypoglossal	

REVIEW QUESTIONS

1. Which structure is not a part of a neuron?
   1. dendrite
   2. cell body
   3. axon
   4. nucleus

2. Which statement by a student nurse reflects correct understanding about neurons?
   1. "The dendrite is a short projection from the cell body that conducts impulses away from the cell body."
   2. "Many axons are covered with a myelin sheath, which is a thick gray substance."
   3. "Cell bodies, most of which are located in the CNS, are clustered in ganglia or nuclei."
   4. "The myelin sheath serves to decrease the speed of nerve impulse conduction in axons and is essential for the survival of larger nerve processes."

3. Which statement about neurotransmitters is false?
   1. The neurotransmitter may be either inhibitory or excitatory.
   2. The inhibitory neurotransmitter is usually acetylcholine (ACh).
   3. Norepinephrine (NE), which may be either excitatory or inhibitory, is another major neurotransmitter.
   4. Neurotransmitters are the chemical messengers of the nervous system.

4. A nurse is evaluating a patient's understanding of the brain. Which statement by the patient indicates a need for further teaching?
   1. "The brain is the control center of the nervous system, generating thoughts, emotions, and speech."
   2. "The left hemisphere has greater control over nonverbal perceptual functions."
   3. "The brain has four major regions: the cerebrum, the diencephalon, the brainstem, and the cerebellum."
   4. "The brain contains four ventricles, which are chambers filled with cerebrospinal fluid (CSF)."

5. Which of the following is not part of the brainstem?
   1. midbrain
   2. pons
   3. medulla oblongata
   4. ventricles

6. The brain contains ventricles, which are chambers filled with cerebrospinal fluid (CSF). How many ventricles are in the brain?
   1. two
   2. three
   3. four
   4. five

7. Which statement about cerebrospinal fluid (CSF) is false?
   1. CFS is a clear and colorless liquid.
   2. CSF forms a cushion for the brain tissue, protects the brain and spinal cord from trauma, helps provide nourishment for the brain, and removes waste products of cerebrospinal cellular metabolism.
   3. The usual amount of cerebrospinal fluid ranges from 20–80 mL and averages about 40 mL.
   4. Cerebrospinal fluid is normally produced and absorbed in equal amounts.

8. Which metabolic factor is the major stimulus for vasodilation, increasing cerebral blood flow?
   1. increased carbon dioxide level
   2. hydrogen ion concentration level
   3. oxygen level
   4. changes in potassium level

9. The spinal cord is surrounded and protected by how many vertebrae?
   1. 13
   2. 23
   3. 33
   4. 43

10. During a patient assessment, the nurse notes that the patient can smile, frown, wrinkle his forehead, show his teeth, puff out his cheeks, purse his lips, raise his eyebrows, and close his eyes against resistance. Which cranial nerve is the nurse assessing?
    1. II
    2. III
    3. V
    4. VII

Nursing Care of Patients with Intracranial Disorders

LEARNING OUTCOMES

1. Compare and contrast the pathophysiology, manifestations, interprofessional care, and nursing care of patients with alterations in level of consciousness and increased intracranial pressure (IICP).
2. Describe criteria for diagnosing persistent vegetative state and brain death.
3. Explain the pathophysiology, manifestations, complications, interprofessional care, and nursing care of intracranial disorders, including seizures, stroke, aneurysms, traumatic brain injury, tumors, and headaches.
4. Discuss the purposes, nursing implications, and health education for the patient and family for medications used to treat intracranial disorders.
5. Discuss surgical options for the treatment of IICP, epilepsy, traumatic brain injury, and brain tumors.

CLINICAL COMPETENCIES

1. Assess the functional status of patients with intracranial disorders and monitor, document, and report abnormal manifestations.
2. Use assessment data, individual and cultural patient values and variations, expressed patient needs and preferences, clinical expertise, and evidence to determine priority nursing diagnoses, and select and implement individualized nursing interventions for patients with intracranial disorders.
3. Administer medications used to treat intracranial disorders knowledgeably and safely.
4. Provide appropriate interventions to patients having intracranial pressure monitoring, tonic-clonic seizures, and intracranial surgery.
5. Effectively communicate with and function within the interprofessional team to plan and provide care of patients with intracranial disorders.
6. Use evidence-based practice to provide care for patients undergoing awake craniotomy.
7. Provide appropriate teaching to facilitate safety and to provide information and support necessary for long-term care of patients with intracranial disorders.
8. Revise the plan of care as needed to provide effective interventions to promote, maintain, or restore functional health status to patients with intracranial disorders.

TERMS MATCHING

Place the letter of the correct definition in the space next to each term.

1. _____ agnosia
2. _____ aphasia
3. _____ apraxia
4. _____ aura
5. _____ brain death
6. _____ cerebral edema
7. _____ concussion
8. _____ consciousness
9. _____ contralateral deficit
10. _____ epidural hematoma
11. _____ epilepsy
12. _____ hemianopia
13. _____ hemiparesis
14. _____ hemiplegia
15. _____ hydrocephalus
16. _____ increased intracranial pressure (IICP)
17. _____ locked-in syndrome
18. _____ neglect syndrome
19. _____ persistent vegetative state (PVS)
20. _____ seizure
21. _____ stroke
22. _____ subdural hematoma
23. _____ transient ischemic attack (TIA)

A. Paralysis of the left or right half of the body

B. An increase in the volume of brain tissue due to abnormal accumulation of fluid in brain cells

C. The cessation and irreversibility of all brain functions, including the brainstem

D. Brief period of localized cerebral ischemia that causes neurologic deficits lasting for less than 24 hours

E. A sustained elevated pressure (≥10 mmHg) in the cranial cavity

F. Defective or absent language function

G. The inability to recognize one or more subjects that were previously familiar

H. Brain injury resulting from a violent jar, shake, or impact with an object

I. To be alert and fully aware of the environment and have intact cognitive abilities but to be unable to communicate through speech or movement because of blocked efferent pathways from the brain

J. Occurs when a stroke on one side of the brain leads to loss or impairment of sensorimotor functions on the opposite site of the body

K. An abnormal accumulation of cerebrospinal fluid within the cerebral ventricles

L. The inability to carry out some motor pattern

M. A sensory-perceptual deficit in which the patient has a disorder of attention

N. A condition in which a person is aware of self and environment and is able to respond appropriately to stimuli

O. A disorder characterized by chronic seizure activity

P. Sensation preceding generalized seizure activity; may be a vague sense of uneasiness or an abnormal sensation

Q. A condition in which neurologic deficits result from a sudden decrease in blood flow to a localized area of the brain

R. A single event of excessive and abnormal electrical discharge

S. Weakness of the left or right half of the body

T. The loss of half of the visual field of one or both eyes

U. A localized mass of blood that collects between the dura mater and the arachnoid mater

V. A collection of blood between the dura mater and the skull

W. A permanent condition of complete unawareness of self and the environment and loss of all cognitive functions

FOCUSED STUDY

1. Discuss medication usage for the treatment of epilepsy. Include discussion about the goals of medication therapy. Also include the action and nursing considerations associated with medications used in the treatment of epilepsy.

_____

_____

_____

_____

_____

2. Discuss the definition of and criteria used for diagnosing brain death.

_____

_____

_____

_____

3. List the five stroke warning signs provided by the Stroke Collaborative (2012).

_____

_____

_____

_____

_____

4. Summarize the purpose and criteria for intracranial pressure (ICP) monitoring.

_____

_____

_____

_____

CASE STUDY

Ashley Smith is an 18-year-old female patient in the emergency room. Ashley's mother tells the nurse that Ashley has been complaining of a headache, nasal congestion, and nausea. Ashley states, "I'm seeing those bright spots again." Answer the following questions based on your knowledge of migraines.

1. Discuss the clinical manifestations of a migraine.

2. What factors are believed to trigger an onset of a migraine?

3. List suggestions to decrease the incidence of migraines.

SHORT ANSWERS

Fill in the table regarding the manifestations of brain tumors by location.

Lobe	Manifestations
Frontal Lobe Tumors	
Parietal Lobe Tumors	
Temporal Lobe Tumors	
Occipital Lobe Tumors	
Cerebellum Tumors	
Pituitary Tumors	

REVIEW QUESTIONS

1. During discharge planning, the nurse is teaching the patient how to decrease incidents of migraine headaches. Which suggestion is incorrect?
   1. Wake up at the same time each morning.
   2. Do not use artificial sweeteners.
   3. Do not consume monosodium glutamate (MSG).
   4. Consume a food source or beverage with caffeine around 6 PM.

2. Doll's eye movements are reflexive movements of the eyes in what direction of head rotation?
   1. opposite
   2. parallel
   3. same
   4. downward

3. Which statement by a student nurse reflects correct understanding about brain death?
   1. "Brain death is the cessation and irreversibility of all brain functions, including the brainstem."
   2. "The exact criteria for establishing brain death are standard from state to state."
   3. "The electrocardiogram (ECG) may be used to establish the absence of cardiac activity when brain death is suspected."
   4. "It is generally agreed that brain death has occurred when there is no evidence of cerebral or brainstem function for 2 to 3 days in a patient who has an abnormal body temperature and is not affected by a depressant drug or alcohol poisoning."

4. If cerebral edema occurs, what happens to intracranial pressure (ICP) and cerebral blood flow (CBF)?
   1. ICP increases, CBF decreases
   2. ICP decreases, CBF increases
   3. ICP increases, CBF increases
   4. ICP decreases, CBF decreases

5. A nurse is planning a seminar about headaches. Which statement on a handout for the seminar needs to be corrected?
   1. Migraine headaches affect about 20 million people in the United States and are more common in women than in men.
   2. There are two types of migraine headaches: common migraine (with an aura) and classic migraine (without an aura).
   3. Migraine headaches are recurring vascular headaches that last from 4–72 hours, often initiated by a triggering event and usually accompanied by a neurologic dysfunction.
   4. The exact causes of migraine are not fully understood, but a relationship exists with serotonin.

6. The nurse is providing first aid to a patient who is having a seizure. Which action should the nurse avoid?
   1. Turn the patient on his side.
   2. Cushion the patient's head.
   3. Place a tongue blade in the patient's mouth.
   4. Loosen items around the patient's neck.

7. During discharge planning, the nurse is teaching the patient's spouse about when she needs to call for medical assistance when her husband is having a seizure. Which statement by the spouse would the nurse correct?
   1. "I will call for help when a seizure lasts over 3 minutes."
   2. "Slow recovery from seizure indicates that I need to call for help."
   3. "If my husband has a second seizure, I will call for assistance."
   4. "If I notice any injuries, I will call for assistance."

8. Which information about hematomas is false?
   1. An epidural hematoma develops in the potential space between the dura and the skull.
   2. Acute subdural hematomas develop over weeks or months.
   3. A subdural hematoma is a localized mass of blood that collects between the dura mater and the arachnoid mater.
   4. Intracerebral hematomas, which may be single or multiple, are associated with contusions.

Nursing Care of Patients with **Spinal Cord Disorders** and **CNS Infections**

LEARNING OUTCOMES

1. Explain the pathophysiology, manifestations, complications, interprofessional care, and nursing care of patients with spinal cord injury, herniated intervertebral disk, spinal cord tumor, and CNS infections.

2. Compare and contrast the pathophysiological effects of injuries and tumors of the spinal cord.

3. Discuss the purposes, nursing implications, and health education of the patient and family for medications used to treat spinal cord injuries, tumors, and CNS infections.

4. Explain the surgical procedures and methods used to stabilize, immobilze, and treat spinal cord injuries.

CLINICAL COMPETENCIES

1. Assess and monitor the functional health status of patients with spinal cord disorders and CNS infections, communicating findings to appropriate interprofessional team members.

2. Demonstrate effective use of individualized and patient-centered strategies as well as evidence-based practice to prioritize care and implement interventions for patients with spinal cord disorders and CNS infections.

3. Adapt individual and cultural values and variations as well as expressed needs and preferences into the plan of care for patients with spinal cord disorders and CNS infections.

4. Administer oral and injectable medications used to treat spinal cord disorders and CNS infections knowledgeably and safely.

5. Provide appropriate and safe care to patients having a carotid endarterectomy, halo fixation, and a posterior laminectomy.

6. Effectively communicate with and function within the interprofessional team to plan and provide care.

7. Utilize assessment data, patient values, and evidence to provide teaching to facilitate self-catheterization, self-care of a ruptured intervertebral disk, and community-based self-care of disabilities resulting from spinal cord disorders and CNS infections.

8. Use evidence-based research to prevent ventilator-associated pneumonia in patients in the neurologic ICU.

9. Revise the plan of care as needed to provide effective interventions to promote, maintain, or restore functional health status to patients with spinal cord disorders and CNS infections.

10. Document care in the electronic medical record and use information management tools to monitor outcomes of care.

11. Particpate in studies and projects to improve the quality and safety of care for patients with spinal cord disorders and CNS infections.

TERMS MATCHING

Place the letter of the correct definition in the space next to each term.

1. _____ autonomic dysreflexia
2. _____ botulism
3. _____ Creutzfeldt-Jakob disease (CJD)
4. _____ diskectomy
5. _____ deformation
6. _____ encephalitis
7. _____ fusion
8. _____ herniation
9. _____ meningitis
10. _____ neurogenic shock
11. _____ paraplegia
12. _____ paresthesia
13. _____ postpoliomyelitis syndrome
14. _____ quadriplegia
15. _____ rabies
16. _____ radiculopathy
17. _____ ruptured intervertebral disk
18. _____ sciatica
19. _____ spinal cord injury (SCI)
20. _____ spinal cord tumor
21. _____ spinal shock
22. _____ tetanus
23. _____ ventilator-associated pneumonia

A. A disorder, also called lockjaw, that is caused by the neurotoxin *Clostridium tetani*

B. An abnormal sensation of the skin, such as numbness, burning, or prickling

C. A complication of a previous infection by the poliomyelitis virus

D. The temporary loss of reflex function (called areflexia) below the level of injury at the cervical and upper thoracic spinal cord

E. An exaggerated sympathetic response that occurs in patients with SCIs at or above the T_6 level

F. Removal of the nucleus pulposus of an intervertebral disk

G. A rapidly progressive, degenerative neurologic disease that causes brain degeneration without inflammation

H. A generalized infection of the parenchyma of the brain or spinal cord

I. A severe, life-threatening form of food poisoning caused by the bacillus *Clostridium botulinum*

J. Inflammation of the meninges of the brain and spinal cord

K. The damage to the neural elements of the spinal cord

L. A condition in which one or more nerves, especially nerve roots, do not function normally

M. Paralysis of the lower portion of the body, sometimes involving the lower trunk

N. Viral (rhabdovirus) infection of the central nervous system transmitted by infected saliva that enters the human body through a bite or an open wound

O. Occurs with damage to the neural structures in the cervical area of the spinal cord, resulting in loss or impairment of motor and/or sensory function in the arms, trunk, legs, and pelvic organs

P. Alteration of the spinal cord and soft tissues caused by abnormal head and body movements

Q. Lumbar back pain that radiates down the posterior leg to the ankle and is increased by sneezing or coughing

R. Insertion of a wedge-shaped piece of bone or bone chips between the vertebrae to stabilize them

S. Occurs when the nucleus pulposus protrudes through a weakened or torn annulus fibrosus of an intervertebral disk

T. Shock resulting from an imbalance between parasympathetic and sympathetic stimulation of vascular smooth muscle

U. Rupture of the cartilage surrounding the intervertebral disk with protrusion of the nucleus pulposus

V. May be benign or malignant, primary or metastatic

W. A preventable secondary complication from intubation and mechanical support

FOCUSED STUDY

1. List the manifestations of spinal shock.

_____
_____
_____
_____
_____

2. Discuss conservative treatment modalities utilized to manage care for a patient with ruptured intervertebral disk.

_____
_____
_____

3. List specific topics to consider during a health history assessment interview of the patient with a spinal cord injury (SCI).

_____
_____
_____
_____
_____

4. Autonomic dysreflexia is an emergency that requires immediate assessment and intervention to prevent complications. Discuss nursing interventions to be implemented should autonomic dysreflexia occur.

_____
_____
_____
_____
_____

CASE STUDY

Sandra Brown is a 25-year-old female who arrived at the emergency department (ED) with a complaint of severe back pain. She has rated her pain a 9/10. Her vital signs were taken upon arrival to the ED and were as follows: B/P = 160/90, HR = 122, RR = 26.

1. In an effort to differentiate the cause of the back injury, what diagnostic tests are anticipated?

2. What medications are used in the management of pain and muscle spasms?

3. What are the goals of conservative treatment if Ms. Brown is diagnosed with a herniated disk?

4. What data will be collected in the health history and physical assessment?

CROSSWORD PUZZLE

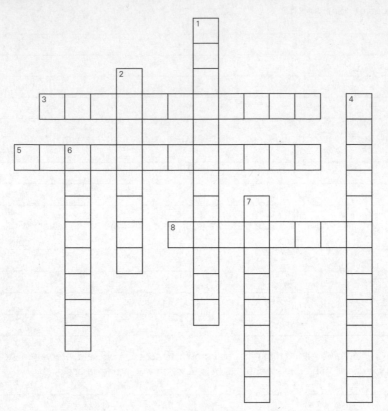

Across

3 Administered to prevent vomiting
5 A forcible bending forward
8 Used to treat bradycardia

Down

1 External force applied in head-on collision
2 A medication used to treat spasticity
4 External force applied in rear-end collision
6 An example of a proton pump inhibitor
7 A medication used to treat hypotension in shock

REVIEW QUESTIONS

1. Which nursing diagosis is the priority for a patient diagnosed with a ruptured intervertebral disk?

   1. *Activity Intolerance*
   2. *Self-Care Deficit*
   3. *Impaired Physical Mobility*
   4. *Acute Pain*

2. Which intervention would not be used when initiating a bowel retraining program?

   1. Assess routine patterns of bowel elimination.
   2. Maintain a high-fluid, low-fiber diet.
   3. Administer stool softeners as prescribed.
   4. Consider implementing manual removal if patient is unable to evacuate.

3. Which findings are clinical manifestations of autonomic dysreflexia? Select all that apply.
   1. hypertension
   2. tachycardia
   3. pounding headache
   4. pallor
   5. nausea

4. During assessment, the nurse would expect which finding in a patient diagnosed with Creutzfeldt-Jakob disease (CJD)?
   1. hyporeflexia
   2. Battle signs
   3. a positive Babinski sign
   4. slowly developing memory changes

5. Which drug is an antifungal agent considered in the treatment of fungal meningitis?
   1. phenytoin (Dilantin®)
   2. amphotericin B (Amphotec®)
   3. rifampin (Rifadin®)
   4. dexamethasone (Decadron®)

6. An emergency department nurse is expected to assess which early manifestation in a patient with tetanus?
   1. stiffness of the jaw and neck
   2. rigidity of abdominal muscles
   3. opisthotonic position
   4. seizure

7. Approximately how much of a fluid loss does a weight loss of 1 lb represent?
   1. 1,500 mL
   2. 1,000 mL
   3. 500 mL
   4. 100 mL

44 Nursing Care of Patients with **Neurologic Disorders**

LEARNING OUTCOMES

1. Identify risk factors for degenerative neurologic, peripheral nervous system (PNS), and cranial nerve disorders.

2. Explain the pathophysiology, manifestations, complications, interprofessional care, and nursing care of patients with degenerative neurologic disorders, PNS disorders, and cranial nerve disorders.

3. Compare and contrast the manifestations of the progressive stages of Alzheimer's disease.

4. Discuss the purposes, nursing implications, and health education for the patient and family for medications used to treat Alzheimer's disease, multiple sclerosis, Parkinson's disease, and myasthenia gravis.

5. Describe the procedures (thymectomy, percutaneous rhizotomy, plasmapheresis) used to treat selected neurologic disorders.

CLINICAL COMPETENCIES

1. Assess and monitor the functional status of patients with neurologic disorders and communicate findings to appropriate interprofessional team members.

2. Demonstrate effective use of individualized and patient-centered strategies as well as evidence-based research to prioritize care and design nursing interventions that are specific to the needs of aging patients with multiple sclerosis.

3. Incoporate assessments, patient needs and preferences (including individual and cultural values), clinical expertise, and evidence-based practice into the formation of priorities and interventions in patients with neurologic disorders.

4. Safely and accurately administer oral and injectable medications used to treat Alzheimer's disease, multiple sclerosis, Parkinson's disease, and myasthenia gravis.

5. Provide competent care to patients having a thymectomy, percutaneous rhizotomy, or plasmapheresis.

6. Effectively communicate with and function within the interprofessional team to plan and provide care of patients with neurologic disorders.

7. Provide appropriate and effective teaching to facilitate safety, communications, and community-based self-care for patients with acute and chronic healthcare needs that result from neurologic disorders.

8. Revise the plan of care as needed to provide effective interventions to promote, maintain, or restore functional health status to patients with neurologic disorders.

9. Document care in the electronic medical record and use information management tools to monitor outcomes of care.

10. Participate in studies and projects to improve the quality and safety of care for patients with neurologic disorders.

TERMS MATCHING

Place the letter of the correct definition in the space next to each term.

1. _____ Alzheimer's disease (AD)
2. _____ amyotrophic lateral sclerosis (ALS)
3. _____ basal ganglia
4. _____ Bell's palsy
5. _____ dementia
6. _____ dopaminergic
7. _____ Guillain-Barré syndrome (GBS)
8. _____ Huntington's disease
9. _____ multiple sclerosis (MS)
10. _____ myasthenia gravis (MG)
11. _____ myelin sheaths
12. _____ neuralgia
13. _____ neurotransmitters
14. _____ Parkinson's disease (PD)
15. _____ trigeminal neuralgia (TN)

A. A chronic autoimmune peripheral nervous system disorder characterized by fatigue and severe skeletal muscle weakness

B. Deeply placed mass of gray matter in the brain; Parkinson's disease is a progressive, degenerative neurologic disorder of these structures

C. An acute inflammatory demyelinating disease of the peripheral nervous system

D. A progressive degenerative neurologic disease characterized by tremor, muscle rigidity, and bradykinesia

E. A form of dementia characterized by progressive, irreversible deterioration of general intellectual functioning

F. A progressive, degenerative inherited neurologic disease characterized by increasing dementia and chorea

G. A chronic demyelinating neurologic disease of the CNS

H. A rapidly progressive and fatal degenerative motor neuron disease characterized by weakness and wasting of voluntary-control muscles but without sensory or cognitive changes

I. A chronic disorder of cranial nerve V that causes severe facial pain

J. A cognitive decline caused by any disorder that permanently damages areas of the brain necessary for memory and learning

K. Nerve pain

L. An acute disorder of cranial nerve VII characterized by unilateral paralysis of the facial muscles

M. A substance or situation that increases the action of dopamine in the brain

N. Fatty, segmented wrappings that normally protect and insulate nerve fibers and increase the speed of nerve impulse transmission

O. A substance (as norepinephrine or acetylcholine) that transmits nerve impulses across a synapse

FOCUSED STUDY

1. Discuss assessment of cranial nerve function and resulting findings.

_____

_____

_____

2. Discuss the criteria that must be met to be diagnosed with dementia and discuss possible risk factors.

_____

_____

_____

_____

3. Summarize the stages of Guillain-Barré syndrome.

_____

_____

_____

_____

4. Describe the following procedures: thymectomy, percutaneous rhizotomy, and plasmapheresis.

_____

_____

_____

_____

_____

CASE STUDY

MiMi Bradley is a 73-year-old female patient in today for a physical examination. Her daughter Christine tells the nurse that her mother has been experiencing memory loss, is having difficulty performing familiar tasks, appears disoriented at times, and is misplacing things, and that she sees a change in her mother's personality. Christine then asks the nurse a few questions. Answer her questions based on your knowledge of Alzheimer's disease.

1. "What are the risk factors of Alzheimer's disease?"

2. "What are the warning signs of Alzheimer's disease?"

3. "What are the stages of Alzheimer's disease?"

WORD SEARCH

C	W	A	S	E	M	D	I	K	G	U	T	P	E	S	H	C	Y	M	J	B
O	E	L	N	O	X	P	O	V	L	D	E	N	B	A	C	L	O	F	E	N
G	S	L	U	N	E	S	A	B	I	R	M	N	M	I	P	W	R	H	T	A
N	Y	Q	B	R	L	F	M	R	W	E	A	V	H	T	A	U	L	F	U	S
L	M	A	T	U	S	T	N	U	L	N	C	E	S	O	I	P	E	I	G	R
A	M	E	R	A	R	A	T	H	P	O	R	N	L	N	A	N	V	N	L	T
I	E	D	M	W	D	L	O	K	Z	A	D	M	M	E	R	I	O	C	Y	M
X	T	U	I	L	S	I	Y	B	F	Q	G	E	T	O	G	V	D	Y	K	H
O	R	S	P	T	S	O	L	A	N	S	A	C	L	S	W	R	O	D	J	C
P	E	I	N	B	W	D	G	V	L	N	C	I	O	D	B	C	P	R	A	T
H	L	X	L	R	E	S	I	R	I	F	K	Y	H	L	F	P	A	Q	L	N
E	M	M	A	U	N	V	M	T	W	A	S	W	O	D	N	S	U	N	C	S
P	R	E	S	J	T	S	N	U	C	L	I	S	M	A	N	Z	E	A	U	J
Z	F	H	Y	O	V	E	T	Y	F	S	E	G	R	D	I	A	D	M	O	A
D	O	N	P	E	G	C	K	A	N	G	H	U	O	L	Y	S	O	N	L	S
E	M	Y	K	O	L	B	T	E	T	D	M	F	S	G	M	B	W	H	R	G
L	M	T	C	N	I	C	M	P	I	I	A	P	R	T	I	O	R	S	Y	O
N	I	U	E	A	P	E	A	R	N	D	E	G	O	Z	A	E	A	J	G	O
J	W	B	S	M	W	K	T	S	O	S	D	I	L	A	N	T	I	N	F	X
Y	D	S	O	A	E	P	K	G	A	Q	Y	N	R	U	W	K	I	C	E	M
S	E	A	C	H	R	I	L	E	H	E	R	W	T	C	L	I	S	N	A	H

DEFINITIONS FOR WORDS IN THE SEARCH

Muscle relaxant	Dopamine agonist	
Immunosuppressant	Anticholinergic	Glucocorticoid
Dopamine precursor	Antiglutamate	
Glutamate antagonist	Anticonvulsant	

REVIEW QUESTIONS

1. Which findings are warning signs of Alzheimer's disease? **Select all that apply.**
   1. habit of misplacing things
   2. loss of initiative
   3. ability to perform familiar tasks
   4. change in personality
   5. withdrawal from social activities

2. Which statement by a student nurse reflects incorrect understanding about multiple sclerosis (MS)? **Select all that apply.**
   1. "It is a chronic demyelinating neurologic disease of the central nervous system."
   2. "The initial onset cannot be followed by a total remission."
   3. "The manifestations of MS do not vary according to the area of the nervous system affected."
   4. "The onset of MS is usually between 40 and 60 years of age."
   5. "It is primarily a disease affecting those of northern European ancestry."

3. During discharge planning, the nurse is teaching the patient about Parkinson's disease. Which statements should be included? **Select all that apply.**
   1. "Parkinson's disease is one of the least common neurologic disorders that affects older adults."
   2. "The disorder usually develops after the age of 75, but 25% of those diagnosed are under 50 years of age."
   3. "Women and men are affected equally."
   4. "Onset of Parkinson's is often subtle."
   5. "Drug-induced Parkinson's is irreversible."

4. Which statement about Parkinson's disease is false?
   1. "In Parkinson's disease, neurons in the cerebral cortex atrophy and are lost, the dopaminergic nigrostriatal (pigmented) pathway degenerates, and the number of specific dopamine receptors in the basal ganglia decreases."
   2. "Diagnosis is based primarily on a thorough history and physical examination and is made based on having one of the three cardinal manifestations: tremor at rest, bradykinesia, and rigidity."
   3. "Surgical treatment of Parkinson's disease may be used for patients who have had the disease for a long time and are no longer able to control manifestations with medications."
   4. "Patients with Parkinson's disease commonly have sleep disturbances, although they may experience decreased manifestations during sleep in the early stages."

5. Which complication is not commonly associated with Parkinson's disease?
   1. falls from balance, posture, and motor changes
   2. depression and social isolation
   3. infections related to immobility
   4. obesity related to dysphagia

6. A nurse is evaluating a patient's understanding of Huntington's disease (HD). Which patient statement indicates a need for further teaching?
   1. "HD is a progressive, degenerative, inherited neurologic disease."
   2. "Early signs of personality change include severe depression."
   3. "Each child of an HD parent has a 25% chance of inheriting the HD gene."
   4. "HD causes destruction of cells in the brain."

7. A nurse is planning a seminar about amyotrophic lateral sclerosis (ALS). Which statement should be included in this discussion?
   1. "ALS is a slow and fatal degenerative neurologic disease."
   2. "ALS is also known as Babe Ruth's disease."
   3. "There is no cure for ALS."
   4. "ALS affects motor neurons in only two locations."

8. The nurse is presenting a class on myasthenia gravis. During the class, she recognizes that further teaching is necessary when which statement is made by a participant?
   1. "Myasthenia gravis is an acute inflammatory demyelinating disorder of the peripheral nervous system."
   2. "The manifestations of myasthenia gravis correspond to the muscles involved."
   3. "In myasthenia gravis, antibodies destroy or block neuromuscular junction receptor sites."
   4. "Myasthenia gravis is sometimes associated with a tumor of the thymus."

9. Which statement by a student nurse reflects incorrect understanding about trigeminal neuralgia? **Select all that apply.**
   1. "Trigeminal neuralgia occurs more commonly in younger adults and affects men more often than women."
   2. "Trigeminal neuralgia is a chronic disease of the trigeminal cranial nerve (V) that causes severe facial pain."
   3. "There are three specific diagnostic tests for trigeminal neuralgia."
   4. "Trigeminal neuralgia is characterized by brief repetitive episodes of sudden severe facial pain."
   5. "Trigeminal neuralgia goes into spontaneous remission for periods lasting from days to years."

Assessing the **Eye** and **Ear**

LEARNING OUTCOMES

1. Describe the anatomy, physiology, and functions of the eye and the ear.
2. Identify specific topics for consideration during a health history interview of the patient with health problems involving the eye or ear.
3. Give examples of genetic disorders in vision and hearing.
4. Describe normal variations in assessment findings for the older adult.
5. Identify abnormal findings that may indicate impairment in the function of the eye and the ear.

CLINICAL COMPETENCIES

1. Conduct and document a health history for patients who have or are at risk for alterations in the structure or functions of the eye and ear, eliciting patient preferences, values, and expressed needs.
2. Safely and effectively assess the structure and functions of the eye and ear, documenting and reporting, as approriate, unexpected findings.
3. Provide appropriate teaching for patients undergoing diagnostic tests of the eyes, ears, vision, or hearing.
4. Monitor the results of diagnostic tests and report abnormal findings.

TERMS MATCHING

Place the letter of the correct definition in the space next to each term.

1. _____ accommodation

2. _____ cerumen

3. _____ convergence

4. _____ corneal reflex

5. _____ hyperopia

6. _____ myopia

7. _____ nystagmus

8. _____ presbyopia

9. _____ presbycusis

10. _____ ptosis

11. _____ pupillary light reflex

12. _____ refraction

A. Farsightedness; the patient is unable to clearly see objects that are near him or her

B. Closure of eyelids (blinking) due to corneal irritation

C. Nearsightedness; the patient is unable to see distant objects well

D. In response to intense light, the pupil normally constricts rapidly

E. The constriction and convergence of the eyes to focus on an object

F. The bending of light rays as they pass from one medium to another medium of different optical density

G. Moving the eyes inward toward the nose to see an object close to the face

H. Age-related impaired near vision resulting from a loss of elasticity of the lens of the eye

I. The brown or yellow waxy substance that is secreted in the ear canal

J. Drooping of one eyelid

K. Rapid involuntary rhythmic movement of the eyes; associated with neurologic disorders and the use of some medications

L. Hearing loss associated with aging

FOCUSED STUDY

1. Identify two nonverbal cues that may indicate that a patient has a problem with his or her eyes.

_____

_____

2. Discuss some age-related changes that can occur in the eye. Discuss some age-related changes that can occur in the ear.

_____

_____

_____

_____

_____

3. Provide three examples of eye disorders that have a genetic influence. Provide three examples of ear disorders that have a genetic influence.

_____

_____

_____

_____

4. Discuss tests that are used to diagnose eye disorders. Discuss tests that are used to diagnose ear disorders.

_____

_____

_____

_____

_____

_____

CASE STUDY

Michael Scott, RN, MSN, is teaching a nursing course. He is preparing a presentation about eye and ear disorders. He has developed the following questions to ask the nursing students after his lecture to evaluate their level of understanding. Use your knowledge of eye and ear disorders to answer these questions.

1. What is the colored part of the eye? What is its function?

2. Where is the lens located? What is its function?

3. What is the best way to assess near vision?

4. How are sound waves transmitted through the ear so that the patient can perceive and interpret the sounds?

5. Explain equilibrium.

6. What is a tympanogram? What does an abnormal tympanogram indicate?

SHORT ANSWERS

1. Identify the following structures: eyebrows, eyelids, eyelashes, conjunctiva, lacrimal apparatus, extrinsic eye muscles. Then compare your answers with Figure 45–1 on page 1474 of your textbook.

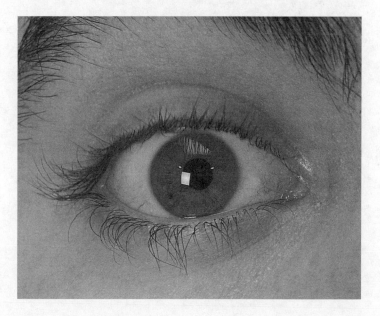

2. Identify the following structures: sclera, cornea, iris, pupil, anterior cavity. Then compare your answers with Figure 45–3 on page 1476 of your textbook.

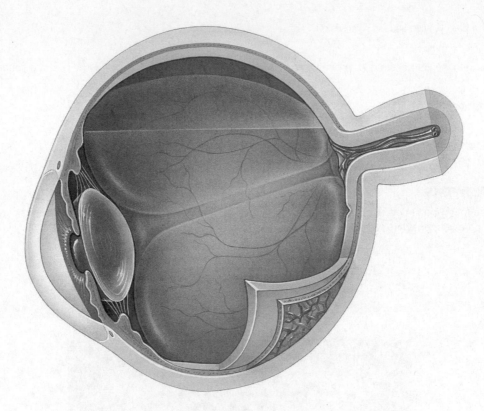

3. Identify the following structures: external ear, middle ear, inner ear. Then compare your answers with Figure 45–10 on page 1483 of your textbook.

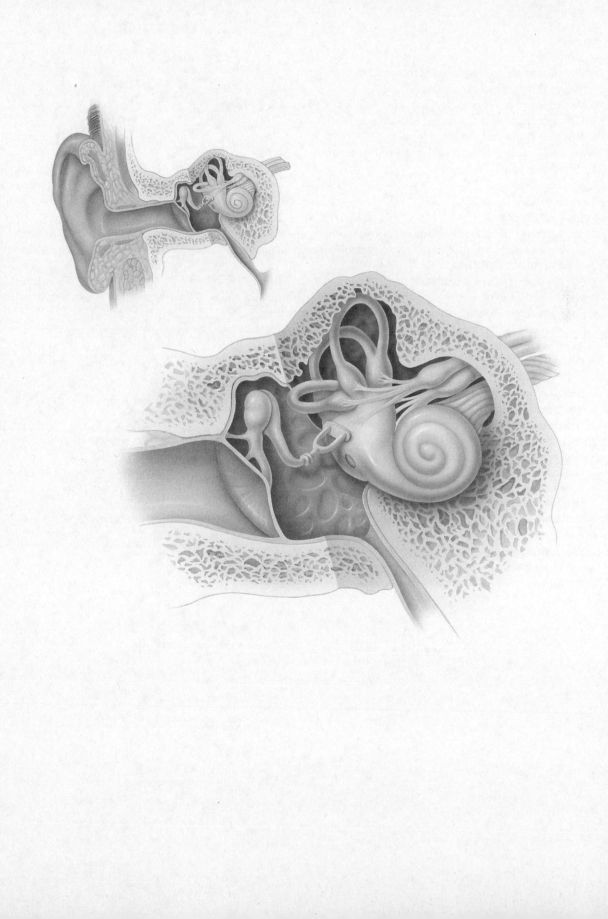

REVIEW QUESTIONS

1. The iris gives the eye its color and regulates light entry by controlling the size of which structure?
  1. pupil
  2. sclera
  3. retina
  4. cornea

2. Which statement about aqueous humor is accurate?
  1. "Aqueous humor is a cloudy fluid."
  2. "Aqueous humor provides nutrients and oxygen to the pupil and the iris."
  3. "The amount of aqueous humor is fixed."
  4. "Aqueous humor fills the anterior cavity."

3. What is the focusing of an image on the retina called?
  1. accommodation
  2. refraction
  3. convergence
  4. pupillary light reflex

4. Which action is correct for the nurse who is measuring a patient's visual fields?
  1. Move the penlight from the periphery toward the center from right to left, above and below, and from the middle of each of these directions.
  2. Ask the patient to look directly at a point behind and to the side of you.
  3. Ask the patient to cover one eye with an opaque cover while you cover your own eye corresponding to the patient's.
  4. Sit directly opposite the patient at a distance of 36–48 inches.

5. Which structure can be found in the external ear?
  1. incus
  2. stapes
  3. malleus
  4. tympanic membrane

6. Which statement about sound conduction indicates the need for further education?
  1. "Hearing is the perception and interpretation of sound."
  2. "Sound is produced when the molecules of a medium are compressed, which results in a pressure disturbance evidenced as a sound wave."
  3. "Sound waves enter the external auditory canal and cause the tympanic membrane to vibrate at the same frequency."
  4. "The human ear is most sensitive to sound waves with frequencies between 100 and 400 cycles per second, but it can detect sound waves with frequencies between 2 and 200 cycles per second."

7. Which assessment finding of the tympanic membrane should be communicated to the patient's physician?
  1. It appears shiny.
  2. The color is pearly gray.
  3. It is translucent.
  4. It is bulging.

Nursing Care of Patients with **Eye** and **Ear Disorders**

LEARNING OUTCOMES

1. Describe the pathophysiology of commonly occurring disorders of the eyes and ears, relating their manifestations and effects on vision and hearing to the pathophysiological process.

2. Explain the risk factors for selected disorders of the eyes and ears, identifying the nursing implications for these risk factors.

3. Identify interprofessional care for specific eye and ear disorders, identifying the nurse's role and responsibilities related to this care.

4. Discuss the effects of and nursing implications for medications prescribed to treat eye and ear disorders.

5. Discuss the nurse's role in caring for patients with impaired vision or hearing loss.

CLINICAL COMPETENCIES

1. Assess the vision, hearing, functional health, and safety of patients with eye and ear disorders, eliciting patient values, preferences, and expressed needs.

2. Using assessment data and current evidence-based practice guidelines, determine priority nursing diagnoses and interventions for patients with eye and ear disorders.

3. Communicate, collaborate, and coordinate with the interprofessional team to provide safe, effective care for patients with eye and ear disorders.

4. Considering patient preferences, values, and expressed needs, plan and implement appropriate and individualized evidence-based nursing interventions and teaching for the patient with an eye or ear disorder.

5. Safely and effectively administer eye and ear medications and prescribed treatments.

6. Critically evaluate the healthcare environment for threats to the safety of patients with eye or ear disorders.

7. Evaluate the effectiveness of care provided for patients with eye and ear disorders, sharing data and revising practices and individual plans of care as indicated.

TERMS MATCHING

Place the letter of the correct definition in the space next to each term.

1. _____ age-related macular degeneration
2. _____ astigmatism
3. _____ cataract
4. _____ conjunctivitis
5. _____ diabetic retinopathy
6. _____ enucleation
7. _____ glaucoma
8. _____ hyperopia
9. _____ hyphema
10. _____ Ménière's disease
11. _____ myopia
12. _____ myringotomy
13. _____ nystagmus
14. _____ otitis media
15. _____ presbycusis
16. _____ ptosis
17. _____ tinnitus
18. _____ tympanoplasty
19. _____ vertigo

A. Inability to see objects in close proximity
B. Inflammation of the middle ear
C. An opacification, or clouding, of the lens of the eye
D. Destructive changes in the macula due to injury or gradual failure of the outer pigmented layer of the retina; affects central vision
E. Rapid involuntary eye movements
F. A chronic disorder characterized by recurrent attacks of vertigo with tinnitus and a progressive unilateral hearing loss; also known as endolymphatic hydrops
G. The surgical reconstruction of the middle ear
H. The perception of a sound such as ringing, buzzing, or roaring in the ears
I. Inflammation of the conjunctiva; the most common eye disease
J. The sensation of movement when there is none; a disorder of equilibrium
K. A vascular disorder that affects the capillaries of the retina
L. Gradual age-related loss of hearing
M. Drooping of the eyelid
N. This develops due to an irregular or abnormal curvature of the cornea; distorts both near and distance vision
O. A condition characterized by optic neuropathy with gradual loss of peripheral vision; often associated with increased intraocular pressure
P. Bleeding in the anterior chamber of the eye
Q. An incision into the tympanic membrane
R. The surgical removal of an eye
S. Inability to see distant objects well

FOCUSED STUDY

1. Identify the various ways that a patient may develop acute conjunctivitis.

_____

_____

_____

_____

2. Explain the difference between nonulcerative and ulcerative keratitis.

_____

_____

_____

3. Briefly describe the tests that can be used to diagnose an inner ear disorder.

_____

_____

_____

4. Discuss the different surgeries that can be performed to correct problems in the patient's ear.

_____

_____

_____

CASE STUDY

Drake Smith is a 21-year-old male patient who is complaining of an itchy right eye. His right eye is red and is draining a small amount of purulent fluid. He was diagnosed with bacterial conjunctivitis. He asks the nurse several questions. Answer his questions based on your knowledge of eye disorders.

1. "Is bacterial conjunctivitis the same as pink eye?"

2. "Is pink eye contagious?"

3. "What do most people with pink eye experience?"

4. "How is it normally treated?"

5. "What are some things I need to know so that I don't give this to my girlfriend?"

6. "My eyes are really sensitive to the sunlight right now. Should I just wear sunglasses until this gets better?"

CARE PLAN CRITICAL-THINKING ACTIVITY

Please refer to the case study and nursing care plan exercise A Patient with Glaucoma and Cataracts in your textbook to answer the following questions.

1. Why is it important for Mrs. Rainey to avoid shutting her eyelids tightly, sneezing, coughing, laughing, bending over, lifting, or straining to have a bowel movement?

2. Why is the red reflex in Mrs. Rainey's right eye diminished on initial assessment?

SHORT ANSWER

Fill in the table regarding the differences between open-angle and angle-closure glaucoma.

	Open-Angle Glaucoma	Angle-Closure Glaucoma
Incidence		
Risk Factors		
Pathophysiology		
Manifestations		
Management		

REVIEW QUESTIONS

1. A patient tells the nurse that he is nearsighted. What does the nurse realize about the patient?

1. The patient is having rapid involuntary eye movements.

2. The patient has an opacification of the lens of the eye.

3. The patient sees objects well at close range but those at a distant are blurred.

4. The patient sees objects better at a distance than objects that are closer.

2. What is a granulomatous cyst or nodule of the lid?

1. hordeolum

2. chalazion

3. hyphema

4. cataract

3. A student nurse is discussing the stages of diabetic retinopathy with an experienced nurse who works with diabetic patients. Which term used by the student nurse indicates that he requires further education?

1. nonproliferative retinopathy

2. background retinopathy

3. proliferative retinopathy

4. dry retinopathy

4. A nurse is evaluating a patient's understanding of otitis externa. Which statement indicates the need for further education?

1. "It is inflammation of the ear canal."

2. "It is commonly known as flyer's ear."

3. "It is most prevalent in people who spend significant time in the water."

4. "Wearing a hearing aid or ear plugs, which hold moisture in the ear canal, is an additional risk factor."

5. Which statement by a student nurse reflects an adequate level of understanding about otosclerosis?

1. "Otosclerosis occurs most commonly in males."

2. "Otosclerosis is not a cause of conductive hearing loss."

3. "Otosclerosis has genetic influences."

4. "Otosclerosis is a hearing loss that typically begins in older patients."

6. Which disorder is chronic and is characterized by recurrent attacks of vertigo with tinnitus and a progressive unilateral hearing loss?

1. acoustic neuroma

2. labyrinthitis

3. Ménière's disease

4. otitis externa

7. A nurse is planning an educational program about presbycusis. Which statement on the handout for the seminar should be corrected?

1. Hearing loss of presbycusis is gradual.

2. Lower-pitched tones and conversational speech are lost initially.

3. It is associated with aging.

4. Hearing aids and other amplification devices are useful for most patients with presbycusis.

LEARNING OUTCOMES

1. Describe the anatomy, physiology, and functions of the male and female reproductive systems, including the breasts.

2. Identify specific topics for consideration during a health history interview of the patient with health problems of the reproductive system and breasts.

3. Give examples of genetic disorders of the male and female reproductive systems and breasts.

4. Describe normal variations in reproductive assessment findings for the older adult.

5. Identify manifestations of impairment in the male and female reproductive systems and breasts.

CLINICAL COMPETENCIES

1. Assess male and female reproductive health status, including physical comfort, values, preferences, and expressed needs.

2. Identify, report, and document normal, abnormal, and unexpected assessments of the male and female reproductive systems.

TERMS MATCHING

Place the letter of the correct definition in the space next to each term.

1. _____ androgens
2. _____ anorgasmia
3. _____ dyspareunia
4. _____ estrogens
5. _____ gynecomastia
6. _____ impotence
7. _____ menstrual cycle
8. _____ menstruation
9. _____ phimosis
10. _____ progesterone
11. _____ semen
12. _____ testosterone

A. Abnormal enlargement of the breast(s) in men

B. Hormones synthesized in the testes, ovaries, and adrenal cortex that promote expression of male sex characteristics

C. The primary androgen produced by the testes that is essential in maintenance of sexual organs and secondary sex characteristics and for spermatogenesis

D. The periodic shedding of the uterine lining in a woman of childbearing age who is not pregnant

E. The inability to achieve or maintain an erection

F. Fluid containing sperm secreted by the male reproductive system glands

G. Hormones produced by the ovaries that are responsible for the normal structure of skin and blood vessels; they also decrease the rate of bone resorption, promote increased high-density lipoproteins, reduce cholesterol levels, and enhance the clotting of blood

H. Cyclic buildup of the uterine lining, ovulation, and sloughing of the lining occurring approximately every 28 days in nonpregnant females of childbearing age

I. A tightness of the prepuce that prevents retraction of the foreskin

J. Failure to achieve an orgasm by intercourse

K. Painful sexual intercourse

L. Hormone produced by the ovaries to support the endometrium in the event of a pregnancy

FOCUSED STUDY

1. Discuss the specific topics for consideration during a health history interview of the patient with health problems involving reproductive and breast structures or functions.

_____
_____
_____
_____
_____

2. Summarize the anatomy and physiology of the female and male reproductive systems.

_____
_____
_____
_____
_____

3. List and explain the functions of the male and female sex hormones.

_____
_____
_____
_____
_____

CASE STUDY

Holly Anne is a 15-year-old female patient. She attended a class about the female reproductive system a few days ago and asks the nurse the following questions. Answer these questions using your knowledge of the female reproductive system.

1. "What are the phases of the menstrual cycle?"

2. "Why do I need estrogen?"

3. "What is the difference between the vagina and the cervix?"

REVIEW QUESTIONS

1. The school nurse is providing a presentation to a group of preteen boys. Which statement about the testes indicates the need for further instruction?
    1. "It is not unusual for one testes to be lower than the other."
    2. "The testes produce sperm and testosterone."
    3. "The testes develop in the abdominal cavity of the fetus and then descend through the spermatic canal into the scrotum."
    4. "The testes are homologous to the female's ovaries."
2. Which statement by a student nurse reflects correct understanding about the prostate gland?
    1. "The prostate gland is about the size of a pea."
    2. "The prostate encircles the urethra just above the urinary bladder."
    3. "The prostate is surrounded by smooth muscle."
    4. "Secretions from the prostate gland make up about two-thirds of the volume of semen."
3. A student nurse is preparing a presentation about the scrotum. Which statement should be corrected prior to the presentation?
    1. "The scrotum is positioned anteriorly to the anus."
    2. "When the testicular temperature is too low, the scrotum contracts to bring the testes up against the body."
    3. "The optimum temperature for sperm production is about 4–5 degrees below body temperature."
    4. "The scrotum hangs at the base of the penis."
4. Which statement by a student nurse reflects correct understanding about female external genitalia?
    1. "The female internal genitalia include the mons pubis, the labia, the clitoris, the vaginal and urethral openings, and glands."
    2. "The clitoris is an erectile organ that is analogous to the penis in the male."
    3. "The labia minora, which are folds of skin and adipose tissue covered with hair, are outermost; they begin at the base of the mons pubis and end at the anus."
    4. "Bartholin and Skene glands have no known sexual purpose."
5. A patient has reported to the physician's office with concerns related to an inability to maintain an erection. The nurse is reviewing the patient's health history. Which medication may be linked to the erectile dysfunction?
    1. antibiotic
    2. oral hypoglycemic agent
    3. antispasmotic
    4. iron supplement
6. Which blood test is used to diagnose prostate cancer and to monitor treatment of prostate cancer?
    1. PSA
    2. VDRL
    3. RPR
    4. FTA-ABS
7. Which female organ(s) is (are) homologous to the male's testes?
    1. fallopian tubes
    2. ovaries
    3. mons pubis
    4. labia minora

48 Nursing Care of **Men** with **Reproductive System** and **Breast Disorders**

LEARNING OUTCOMES

1. Explain the pathophysiology, manifestations, complications, interprofessional care, and nursing care of disorders of the male reproductive system, including disorders of sexual function, the penis, the testes and scrotum, the prostate gland, and the breast.

2. Compare and contrast the risk factors for cancer of the penis, testes, and prostate gland.

3. Discuss the purposes, nursing implications, and health education for medications and treatments used to treat disorders of sexual function, the penis, the testes and scrotum, the prostate gland, and the breast.

4. Describe the various surgical procedures used to treat disorders of the male reproductive system.

CLINICAL COMPETENCIES

1. Assess the functional health status of men with reproductive system and breast disorders and monitor, document, and report abnormal manifestations and responses.

2. Use current evidence and patient preferences to plan and implement optimal nursing care for men with reproductive and breast disorders.

3. Prompt patient responses of values, preferences, and expressed needs as part of the clinical interview, implementation, and evaluation of care.

4. Function competently within own scope of practice as a member of the healthcare team caring for men with reproductive and breast disorders.

5. Apply quality measures, processes, and tools to improve outcomes for men with or at risk for reproductive and breast disorders.

TERMS MATCHING

Place the letter of the correct definition in the space next to each term.

1. _____ benign prostatic hyperplasia (BPH)
2. _____ epididymitis
3. _____ erectile dysfunction (ED)
4. _____ gynecomastia
5. _____ hydrocele
6. _____ impotence
7. _____ libido
8. _____ orchitis
9. _____ phimosis
10. _____ premature ejaculation
11. _____ priapism
12. _____ prostatitis
13. _____ retrograde ejaculation
14. _____ spermatocele
15. _____ testicular torsion
16. _____ varicocele

A. The inability of the male to attain and maintain an erection sufficient to permit satisfactory sexual intercourse

B. Inability to achieve or maintain an erection

C. A term used to describe sexual desire

D. An age-related, nonmalignant enlargement of the prostate gland that begins at 40–45 years of age and continues slowly through the rest of life

E. An abnormal and often painful dilation of the pampiniform venous complex in the spermatic cord caused by incompetent or congenitally missing valves that allow blood to pool in the spermatic cord veins

F. Sustained, painful erection that lasts at least 4 hours and is not associated with sexual arousal

G. Constriction of the foreskin so that it cannot be retracted over the glans penis

H. The discharge of seminal fluid into the urinary bladder that may develop in aging men but is usually related to treatment of prostate conditions or testicular cancer

I. Inflammatory disorders of the prostate gland

J. An infection or inflammation of the epididymis, the structure that lies along the posterior border of the testis

K. The twisting of the testes and spermatic cord resulting in sudden onset of scrotal swelling, pain, and nausea and vomiting; it occurs most often between birth and age 20 but can occur at any age

L. A mobile, usually painless mass containing dead spermatozoa that forms in the epididymis

M. The abnormal enlargement of the male breast thought to result from a high ratio of estradiol to testosterone

N. A common ejaculatory disorder in which semen is ejaculated before completion of sexual intercourse

O. The collection of fluid in the tunica vaginalis

P. An acute inflammation or infection of the testes

FOCUSED STUDY

1. List the risk factors for cancer of the penis, testes, and prostate gland.

_____

_____

_____

2. Summarize the various surgical procedures used to treat disorders of the male reproductive system.

_____

_____

_____

3. List the diagnostic tests that may be used to assess the patient who is reporting erectile dysfunction. Once the testing is completed, what treatment options are available to manage this condition?

_____

_____

_____

CASE STUDY

Nathaniel Obermark is a 22-year-old male patient who states, "I have slight enlargement of my right testicle with some discomfort, and I have a feeling of heaviness in the scrotum." He then asks the nurse the following questions. Answer the questions based on your knowledge of the male reproductive system.

1. "What is the cause of testicular cancer?"

2. "What are the risk factors for testicular cancer?"

3. "What are the manifestations of testicular cancer?"

SHORT ANSWERS

Complete the chart by indicating the appropriate cause of erectile dysfunction for each category.

Medications	Procedures	Neurogenic Causes	Arterial Causes
1.	1.	1.	1.
2.	2.	2.	2.
3.	3.	3.	3.
4.	4.	4.	4.
5.	5.	5.	
6.	6.	6.	
7.	7.		
	8.		
	9.		
	10.		

REVIEW QUESTIONS

1. The nurse is providing a program about erectile dysfunction. When he is assessing the knowledge level of the participants, which statement indicates the need for further education?
   1. "Erectile dysfunction is the male's inability to attain and maintain an erection sufficient to permit satisfactory sexual intercourse."
   2. "*Impotence* is a term often used synonymously with *erectile dysfunction*."
   3. "Erectile dysfunction has many possible causes."
   4. "Erectile dysfunction can be treated only with oral medications."

2. Which condition is constriction of the foreskin so that it cannot be retracted over the glans penis?
   1. paraphimosis
   2. phimosis
   3. priapism
   4. hydrocele

3. What is a collection of fluid in the tunica vaginalis and is the most common cause of scrotal swelling?
   1. testicular torsion
   2. spermatocele
   3. hydrocele
   4. varicocele

4. Which statement by a student nurse reflects correct understanding about orchitis?
   1. "Orchitis is a chronic infection of the testes."
   2. "Orchitis most commonly occurs as a complication of a systemic illness or as an extension of epididymitis."
   3. "The most common infectious cause of orchitis in postpubertal men is measles."
   4. "Sterility from orchitis is rare."

5. A nurse is evaluating a patient's understanding of testicular cancer. Which statement indicates a need for further teaching?
   1. "Testicular cancer is more common on the left side."
   2. "Testicular cancer is the most common cancer in men between the ages of 15 and 40."
   3. "The first sign of testicular cancer may be a slight painless enlargement of one testicle."
   4. "Testicular cancer is more common on the right side, which parallels the incidence of cryptorchidism."

6. A nurse is planning a seminar about benign prostatic hyperplasia (BPH). Which statement on an educational handout should be corrected?
   1. The two necessary preconditions for BPH are age of 48 and older and the presence of testes.
   2. BPH, which is the twisting of the spermatic cord with scrotal swelling and pain, is a potential medical emergency.
   3. The exact cause of BPH is unknown.
   4. Risk factors of BPH include age, family history, race, and a diet high in meat and fats.

7. What is a mobile, usually painless mass that forms when efferent ducts in the epididymis dilate and form a cyst?
   1. spermatocele
   2. testicular torsion
   3. hydrocele
   4. varicocele

8. A patient has reported to the clinic with manifestations consistent with epididymitis. When assisting the physician, the nurse recognizes that the condition will likely be diagnosed using which test?
   1. urethral swab culture
   2. blood cultures
   3. ultrasound
   4. urinalysis

CHAPTER 49

Nursing Care of **Women** with **Reproductive System** and **Breast Disorders**

LEARNING OUTCOMES

1. Explain the pathophysiology, manifestations, complications, interprofessional care, and nursing care of disorders of female sexual function, menstrual disorders, structural disorders, reproductive tissue disorders, and breast disorders.

2. Describe the physiologic process of perimenopause.

3. Compare and contrast the incidence, risk factors, pathophysiology, manifestations, diagnosis, treatment, and nursing care for cancer of the cervix, endometrium, ovary, vulva, and breast.

4. Explain the purposes, nursing implications, and health education for women and their families for cancer screening, medications, and treatments for disorders of the reproductive system and breast.

5. Discuss alternative and complementary therapies used by women to relieve manifestations associated with menopause and menstrual disorders.

6. Describe the surgical procedures used to treat female reproductive system and breast disorders.

CLINICAL COMPETENCIES

1. Assess the functional health status of women with reproductive system and breast disorders and monitor, document, and report abnormal manifestations and responses.

2. Use current evidence and patient preferences to plan and implement optimal nursing care for women with reproductive and breast disorders.

3. Prompt patient responses of values, preferences, and expressed needs as part of the clinical interview, implementation, and evaluation of care.

4. Function competently within own scope of practice as a member of the healthcare team caring for women with reproductive and breast disorders.

5. Apply quality measures, processes, and tools to improve outcomes for women with or at risk for reproductive and breast disorders.

TERMS MATCHING

Place the letter of the correct definition in the space next to each term.

1. _____ amenorrhea

2. _____ anorgasmia

3. _____ dysfunctional uterine bleeding (DUB)

4. _____ dysmenorrhea

5. _____ dyspareunia

6. _____ endometriosis

7. _____ fibrocystic changes (FCC)

8. _____ leiomyoma

9. _____ lymphedema

10. _____ menopause

11. _____ menorrhagia

12. _____ metrorrhagia

13. _____ premenstrual syndrome (PMS)

A. A condition in which a woman has never experienced an orgasm during the waking state, either through self-stimulation or intercourse

B. Bleeding between menstrual periods that may be caused by hormonal imbalances, pelvic inflammatory disease, cervical or uterine polyps, uterine fibroids, or cervical or uterine cancer

C. Benign tumors that originate from smooth muscle of the uterus and are referred to as fibroid tumors

D. The permanent cessation of menses as a result of aging, surgical removal of the ovaries, or chemotherapy

E. Painful sexual intercourse

F. Edema of an extremity due to accumulated lymph; may be primary or secondary, resulting from inflammation, obstruction, or removal of lymphatic vessels

G. The absence of menstruation

H. The physiological nodularity and breast tenderness that increases and decreases with the menstrual cycle and is experienced by an estimated 50–80% of all women

I. A complex of manifestations (e.g., mood swings, breast tenderness, fatigue, irritability, food cravings, and depression) that are limited to 3–14 days before menstruation and relieved by the onset of menses

J. Vaginal bleeding that is usually painless but abnormal in amount, duration, or time of occurrence

K. Excessive or prolonged menstruation that may result from thyroid disorders, endometriosis, pelvic inflammatory disease, functional ovarian cysts, or uterine fibroids or polyps

L. Pain or discomfort associated with menstruation that is estimated to occur in 46–95% of menstruating women

M. A condition in which multiple, small implants of endometrial tissue develop throughout the pelvic cavity

FOCUSED STUDY

1. List alternative and complementary therapies used by women to relieve manifestations associated with menopause and menstrual disorders.

_____

_____

_____

_____

2. Summarize the surgical procedures used to treat female reproductive system disorders.

_____

_____

_____

3. Discuss the physiological process of menopause.

_____

_____

_____

4. List the risk factors, manifestations, and treatment for cancer of the cervix.

_____

_____

_____

_____

CASE STUDY

Elizabeth Baldwin is a 21-year-old female patient. She is in today to have her first Pap test and breast examination. Answer the following questions based on your knowledge of Pap tests and breast examinations.

1. How often does the American Cancer Society recommend that women have Pap tests?

2. Is Elizabeth a good candidate to receive Gardasil®? Why or why not?

3. What are the instructions for performing a breast self-examination?

CROSSWORD PUZZLE

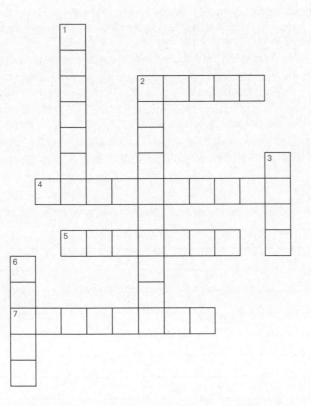

Across

2 Vascular solid tumor attached by a pedicle

4 Tumor removal leaving the uterus intact

5 Abnormal opening between two organs

7 Vaccine administered to prevent cervical cancer as a result of HPV

Down

1 Removable device used to support the uterus

2 Progesterone-like medications

3 Fluid-filled sac

6 Exercises used to strengthen pelvic muscles

REVIEW QUESTIONS

1. A nurse is leading a seminar about menopause. Which statement made by a participant is correct?
1. "Menopause is a disease and is not a normal physiological process."
2. "Menopause is the permanent cessation of menses."
3. "Late menopause is associated with genetics, smoking, higher altitude, and obesity."
4. "The average woman will live one-fourth of her life after menopause."

2. The nurse is taking the health history of a woman who has come to the physician's office with reproductive-related concerns. During the health history, the woman reveals that she has been experiencing bleeding between menstrual periods. What term should be documented by the nurse?
1. menorrhagia
2. metrorrhagia
3. oligomenorrhea
4. amenorrhea

3. During a pelvic examination, the physician explains to the nurse that the patient's uterus is tilting forward in an exaggerated manner. What term can the nurse expect the physician to use to refer to this condition?
1. retroversion
2. retroflexion
3. anteversion
4. anteflexion

4. A nurse is evaluating a patient's understanding of breast self-examination (BSE). Which statement indicates a need for further teaching?
1. "Lie down on your back and place your right arm behind your head."
2. "Use three different levels of pressure to feel all of the breast tissue."
3. "Use overlapping quarter-sized circular motions of the finger pads to feel the breast tissue."
4. "Look at your breasts for any changes in size, shape, contour, or dimpling."

5. A nurse is conducting a seminar about ovarian cancer. Which statement by a participant indicates understanding?
1. "Ovarian cancer is the most common gynecologic cancer in women in the United States."
2. "An enlarged abdomen with ascites signals early-stage disease."
3. "There are several types of ovarian cancers: epithelial tumors, germ cell tumors, and gonadal stromal tumors."
4. "In early stages, ovarian cancer generally causes several warning signs or manifestations."

6. A nurse is evaluating a patient's understanding of fibrocystic changes (FCC), or fibrocystic breast disease. Which statement indicates a need for further teaching?
1. "FCC is the physiological nodularity and breast tenderness that increases and decreases with the menstrual cycle."
2. "FCC is most common in women 20–30 years of age and is common in postmenopausal women who are not taking hormone replacement."
3. "FCC includes many different lesions and breast changes."
4. "Women with fibrocystic changes experience bilateral or unilateral pain or tenderness in the upper, outer quadrants of their breasts and report that their breasts feel particularly thick and lumpy the week prior to menses."

7. A nurse is planning an educational program about premenstrual syndrome (PMS). When preparing the handout, which statement may be correctly included?
1. PMS is never a factor in absenteeism at school or work, decreased productivity, difficulties in interpersonal relationships, and disruption in lifestyle.
2. Manifestations of PMS occur during the follicular phase of the menstrual cycle (3–6 days prior to the onset of the menstrual flow) and abate when the menstrual flow begins.
3. The treatment of PMS integrates a self-monitored record of manifestations, regular exercise, caffeine, and a diet low in simple sugars and lean proteins.
4. Alternative and complementary therapies that the woman with PMS may find helpful focus on diet, exercise, relaxation, and stress management.

8. What kind of uterine prolapse is complete prolapse of the uterus outside the body, with inversion of the vaginal canal?
1. mild
2. first degree
3. second degree
4. third degree

50 Nursing Care of Patients with **Sexually Transmitted Infections**

LEARNING OUTCOMES

1. Explain the incidence, prevalence, characteristics, and prevention/control of sexually transmitted infections (STIs).
2. Compare and contrast the pathophysiology, manifestations, interprofessional care, and nursing care of genital herpes, genital warts, vaginitis, chlamydia, gonorrhea, syphilis, and pelvic inflammatory disease.
3. Explain the risk factors for and complications of STIs.
4. Discuss the effects and nursing implications of medications and treatments used to treat STIs.

CLINICAL COMPETENCIES

1. Assess the functional health status of patients with STIs and monitor, document, and report abnormal manifestations.
2. Determine priority nursing diagnoses and select and implement evidence-based and patient-centered nursing interventions for patients with STIs.
3. Administer topical, oral, and injectable medications knowledgeably and safely.
4. Integrate interprofessional care into care of patients with STIs.
5. Provide teaching appropriate for prevention, control, and self-care of STIs.
6. Revise the plan of care as needed to provide effective interventions to promote, maintain, or restore functional health status to patients with STIs.

TERMS MATCHING

Place the letter of the correct definition in the space next to each term.

1. _____ chancre

2. _____ chlamydia

3. _____ dyspareunia

4. _____ gonorrhea

5. _____ pelvic inflammatory disease (PID)

6. _____ sexually transmitted infections (STIs)

7. _____ syphilis

A. A painless, hard, syphilitic primary ulcer

B. Infections transmitted by vaginal, oral, and anal intimate contact and intercourse

C. Painful sexual intercourse

D. A bacterial infection that may be asymptomatic for an extended period of time after infection; it typically involves the cervix in women and the urethra in men

E. A complex systemic STI caused by the spirochete *Treponema pallidum*; it can infect almost any body tissue or organ and is transmitted from open lesions during any sexual contact (genital, oral–genital, or anal–genital)

F. An infection of the pelvic organs, including the fallopian tubes (salpingitis), ovaries (oophoritis), cervix (cervicitis), endometrium (endometritis), pelvic peritoneum, and pelvic vascular system

G. The most commonly reported sexually transmitted infection; it is bacterial in nature and often is referred to as the "clap"

FOCUSED STUDY

1. Explain the nursing implications of medications and treatments used to treat sexually transmitted infections.

_____

_____

2. List the information essential to an accurate sexual history.

_____

_____

3. Discuss the interprofessional care and nursing care of sexually transmitted infections.

_____

_____

_____

_____

_____

4. Summarize the prevention/control of sexually transmitted infections.

_____

_____

CASE STUDY

A 21-year-old patient is seen at the family planning clinic with complaints consistent with a genital herpes simplex infection. During the nurse's interaction with the patient, the patient asks several questions. Answer the following questions based on your knowledge of sexually transmitted infections.

1. "What causes genital herpes?"

2. "How will this be cured?"

3. "What happens with the virus between outbreaks?"

4. "How long will it take for the related symptoms to go away?"

SHORT ANSWERS

Fill in the table regarding sexually transmitted diseases.

Infection	Characteristics of Discharge
Candidiasis	
Bacterial vaginosis.	
Trichomoniasis	
Gonorrhea	

REVIEW QUESTIONS

1. Sexually transmitted infections (STIs) have reached epidemic proportions in the United States and continue to increase worldwide. Which statement about STIs is incorrect?
   1. Many STIs are more easily transmitted from a woman to a man than from a man to a woman.
   2. The incidence of STIs is highest in young adults aged 15–24.
   3. STIs are caused by bacteria, *Chlamydiae*, viruses, fungi, protozoa, and parasites.
   4. Infections that are transmitted by vaginal, oral, and anal intimate contact and intercourse are referred to as sexually transmitted infections (STIs).

2. What is associated with cold sores but may be transmitted to the genital area by oral intercourse or by self-inoculation through poor handwashing practices?
   1. HSV-2
   2. HPV
   3. HSV-1
   4. GC

3. Which of these diseases is not a reportable disease?
   1. genital warts
   2. gonorrhea
   3. syphilis
   4. AIDS

4. When preparing to discuss chlamydia with a patient, the nurse recognizes which statement to be incorrect?
   1. "Because chlamydia is asymptomatic in most women until the uterus and fallopian tubes have been invaded, treatment may be delayed, which results in devastating long-term complications."
   2. "Chlamydia typically invades cells of the urethra in both sexes."
   3. "The infections caused by chlamydia include acute urethral syndrome, nongonococcal urethritis, mucopurulent cervicitis, and pelvic inflammatory disease (PID)."
   4. "Complications of chlamydial infections in men include epididymitis, prostatitis, sterility, and Reiter's syndrome."

5. What stage of syphilis is characterized by the appearance of a chancre and by regional enlargement of the lymph nodes with little or no pain accompanying these warning signs?
   1. secondary
   2. latent
   3. primary
   4. tertiary

6. A nurse is planning a seminar about pelvic inflammatory disease (PID). Which statement on an educational handout should be corrected?
   1. PID is a reportable disease in the United States.
   2. PID is usually polymicrobial (caused by more than one microbe) in origin; gonorrhea and chlamydia are common causative organisms.
   3. Manifestations of PID include fever, purulent vaginal discharge, severe lower abdominal pain, and a painful cervical movement.
   4. Complications include pelvic abscess, infertility, ectopic pregnancy, chronic pelvic pain, pelvic adhesions, and dyspareunia. Abscess formation is common.

7. Which of the following are slightly raised lesions that are often invisible to the naked eye and develop on keratinized skin?
    1. keratotic warts
    2. papular warts
    3. flat warts
    4. condyloma acuminata
8. Which statement by a student nurse reflects an accurate understanding of trichomoniasis?
    1. "It is caused by *Trichomonas vaginalis,* a protozoan parasite."
    2. "It is the least common noncurable STI in young, sexually active women."
    3. "Manifestations of trichomoniasis usually appear within 1 to 4 days of exposure."
    4. "Women with trichomoniasis have a nonfrothy, red-orange vaginal discharge with a strong fishy odor that is often accompanied by itching and irritation of the genitalia."